KETOGENIC DIET

Ketogenic Diet for Weight Loss

14 Day Ketogenic Weight Loss Meals Plans

PLUS 21 Delicious Ketogenic Recipes to Keep You Burning Fat and Staying Healthy All Day Long!

BONUS Ketogenic Recipes for Breakfast, Lunch and Dinner! Even Ketogenic Shakes!

VALERIE CHILDS

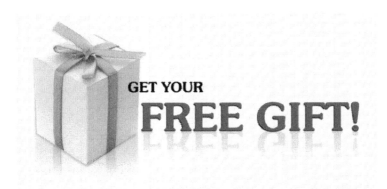

GET YOUR

FREE GIFT!

WAIT! – DO YOU LIKE FREE BOOKS?

My **FREE Gift** to You!! As a way to say **Thank You** for downloading my book, I'd like to offer you more **FREE BOOKS!** Each time we release a NEW book, we offer it first to a small number of people as a test - drive. Because of your commitment here in downloading my book, I'd love for you to be a part of this group. You can join easily here → http://www.fatlosswithpaleo.com

Table of Contents

Preface

"You're going to go through tough times - that's life. But I say, 'Nothing happens to you, it happens for you'. See the positive in negative events"

- Joel Osteen

"A life spent making mistakes is not only more honorable, but more useful than a life spent doing nothing"

- George Bernard Shaw

This eBook aims at helping those individuals yearning to live a healthy life. In the modern world, the everyday upheavals are pronounced. While few of us are able to cope up with these stressful conditions, few of us end up developing habits that we later regret for having done. It is during this period when we try to reverse the damage we have causes to ourselves and our self esteem.

Binge eating or eating disorder can lead to unhealthy eating habits, the consequences of which can be fatal and disappointing.

Given the fact that there are a number of crash diets doing their rounds in the market these days, here we will like to introduce and enlighten you with the ketogenic diet plan.

As experts have said that this form of diet is a "powerful tool" that can help you to wriggle out of a number of diseases and ailments, the consequences of which lead to despair among the ones suffering.

Chapter 1

THE BASICS

Understanding Ketogenic Diet

A ketogenic diet is also known as keto diet. It is basically a low carbohydrate diet, wherein ketones are produced by the liver so that the same is used as energy. The other short form of this diet is LCHF or Low carb high fat diet. Whenever there is intake of high carbohydrate dishes, there will be production of insulin as well as glucose. Generally, glucose is used as energy source for all our activities. And when it comes to insulin, its production processes the glucose that is produced in the bloodstream when there is high intake of carbohydrate. This glucose is processed and distributed throughout the body. So, it is seen that the role of fat in the production of energy is negligible or in other words, absolutely unnecessary, when it comes as the primary source of energy. Whenever, carbohydrate intake is restricted, a condition known as ketosis is induced. It is a naturally occurring process, wherein ketones are produced in the liver as a result of breakdown of fat.

The main aim of ketogenic diet is to inculcate this kind of metabolic state in the body. And this is essentially achieved not by compromising on the calories but by compromising on carbohydrate intake.

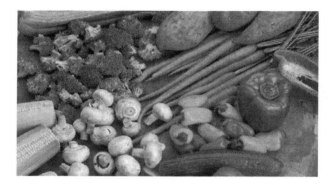

Intro into Keto adaptation

Unlike the normal process, wherein glucose is used as the primary source of energy, as you shift to ketogenic diet, your body starts getting accustomed to fat metabolism. This shift is quite crucial and involves most of the organs of the body like kidney, muscles, brain, and liver. So, it has been generally observed that the body is able to get into a state of ketosis very easily but when it comes to keto adaptation, the process is quite complex. Keto adaptation is ideal for people that do not regard as this diet plan as a short term tool of weight loss but adopt it as a lifestyle change where there is low intake of carbohydrate. The time taken by the body to adapt to the new state of metabolism usually differs from one individual to another and it may be between 3 weeks and 4 weeks or even for months that the body takes to get into the state of ketosis.

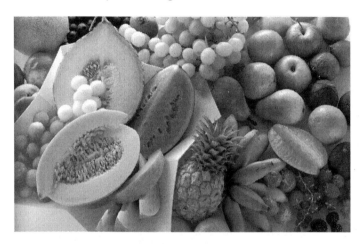

Effect of Keto diet on the body

Generally, our bodies are used to using up carbohydrates as the primary source of energy. Ever since we are born, over the years as we evolve, there are certain specific enzymes that play an instrumental role in the breakdown of fat in the body. When the state of ketosis is induced, the body has to deal with the sudden change. There is glucose insufficiency and there is build up of fat in the body. Also, a new set of enzymes build over a period of time to acclimatize to the new changes that take place in the body. As a result, if there is less intake of carbohydrate, the body will naturally use up the left over glucose present in the body. As a result there is depletion of glycogen in the body, which may lead to feeling of general lethargy. So, in the initial stages, if you have taken to ketogenic diet, you may company about confusion, headaches, feeling dizzy, flu-like symptoms, and irritability. In other words, it is quite likely that you might have symptoms resemble that of PMS or premenstrual symptoms.

All these symptoms usually take place due to flushing out of electrolytes from the body. Ketosis instills diuretic effects in the body. In order to prevent yourself from dehydration, it is important o stay hydrated at all times adequately. Also, the sodium intake should be maintained. Salt intake should be increased to a certain extent. This will not starve you of the electrolytes and the same will be replenished from time to time.

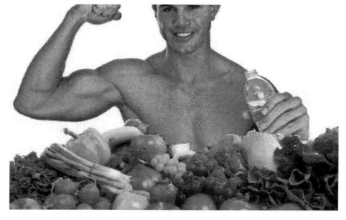

Benefits you can count on

The introduction of ketogenic diet leads to a state called ketosis. The benefits are manifold and these can be enumerated as below-

✓ **Hypoglycemia** - One of the best advantages of switching over to ketogenic diet is that the condition of hypoglycemia can be controlled to a great extent. Also, unlike other times, when sugar cravings are pronounced when you are not on ketogenic diet, this problem can be addressed easily when you switch over to keto diet.

✓ **Hunger pangs** - When you start keto diet, you don't get hunger pangs easily. In fact, it can be safely said that your appetite is lost. As a result, your cravings for food are also reduced greatly. There are several instances when individuals have complained that even if they have skipped a meal, they did not feel as if they have not eaten anything.

✓ **Mood stabilizer** - Ketone bodies that are formed in as a result of ketosis helps in stabilizing the neurotransmitters. Serotonin and dopamine are essentially worked upon, which contributes to the mood enhancement feeling in an individual that has taken up the ketogenic diet.

✓ **Aids digestion**- If you have trouble in digesting food it improves gut health.

✓ **Relief from heartburn** - Individuals suffering from GERD can heave a sigh of relief as these symptoms disappear fully. It has been observed that people taking grains and sugar based food items at night are prone to heartburn. So, eliminating sugar or having less sugar in the body helps you to do away with the problem of heartburn or GERD.

✓ **Gum related ailments** - People fond of sweets and sugar based goodies are susceptible to gum diseases as the pH of the mouth changes remarkably. If you can continue ketogenic diet plan for a period of 3 and 4 months, you will notice that you have got rid of any tooth problem you had before like tooth decay and gum inflammation.

✓ **Weight loss** - One of the greatest achievements of switching over to ketogenic diet is that you can enjoy effective weight loss. However, it has been observed that individuals that suffer from insulin resistance and have a considerably high fasting sugar in blood have to complement the ketogenic diet with regular appropriate exercises as suggested by an expert trainer.

✓ **Boost in energy**- Keto-flu is a phenomenon that many people opting for ketognic diet might complain of in the initial stages of the introduction of the diet. It is also known as 'low carb flu'. But if you are able to overcome this phase, rest assured that you will feel great and rejuvenated thereafter.

✓ **Better managed blood pressure** - If you are used to eating high carbohydrate food items, over a period of time, you will find out that your blood pressure is gradually escalating. However, for the effective control of blood pressure, switch over to ketogenic diet, which controls blood pressure in a remarkable manner. It might also happen that your GP will suggest that you reduce the number of medicines you are taking to control blood pressure.

✓ **Better control over cholesterol** - Eating sugar-rich food items might adversely affect your arterial system as cholesterol comprises excess sugar. And if you have developed the habit of consuming less sugar based food items, you can be assured that your cholesterol will also be remarkably controlled.

✓ **Improved hbA1c and CRP** - Adopting keto diet will help you by allowing you to have better readings in hbA1c and CRP levels. These are regarded as markers that indicate whether or not your general well being is adversely affected.

✓ **Triglyceride readings improve** - One of the most significant achievements of adopting ketogenic diet is that as the carbohydrate level of consumption is minimized, the triglyceride levels also drop significantly. Triglyceride level :

HDL is a marker of heart disease and should be monitored carefully at regular intervals.

✓ **Clearer thought process** - There are times when our thought process becomes hazy and we are not clear about our objectives and goals. It is during this phase that we tend to suffer from depression, anxiety, and tend to imbibe all negative thoughts. This negative attitude is reflected in our behavior and health. If you have adopted keto diet, it won't be long when you will have a better mind set and better ability to take decisions and judge.

✓ **Better sleep patterns** - Studies and research has also proved that with this kind of diet plan, there was marked improved in sleep patterns in individuals that had problems in sleeping and the ones that suffered from problems related to sleep apnea.

✓ **Improved joint coordination** - As we grow older or if we strain our muscles and joints too much, it is quite likely that we end up injuring ourselves and eventually the joints become stiff and pain. You can do away with these troubles if you start living on keto diet.

It takes just a couple of weeks when you can actually see the results. So, when you have the provision to lead a better life, why not try out this new approach and alternative method of getting rid of all the ailments that have crippled you all these years and restricted you from leading a healthy life.

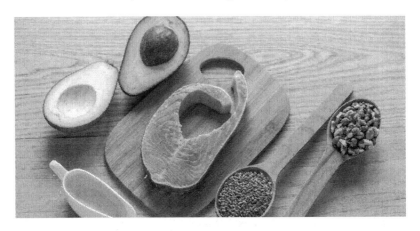

Drawbacks to watch out for

Ketogenic diet, we know comprises low carb and high fat diet. It leads into a state called ketosis. This form of diet aids in addressing several health related problems as mentioned above. However, experts are of the opinion and studies have also proved that if you consume high fat diet and a low carbohydrate diet over a prolonged period of time, it can have damaging effects on the body in the long run.

✓ **Prone to heart disease** - There few categories of high fat food items that include egg yolks, coconut, and lard. These have a high saturated fat content but low carbohydrate as well as protein content. Consuming this kind of food over a long period of time makes you susceptible to heart diseases. Also, it has been observed that diet high in fat content have detrimental effect on the brain cells. This is because there is a set of brain cells that regulate body weight.

✓ **Effect on liver and muscles** - Carbohydrate is stored in our bodies mainly in the liver and muscles in the form of glycogen. An individual requires approximately 600 calories to sustain daily without eating anything. But if you are not into too much of exercising and have been leading a sedentary life most time of your life, the carbohydrate starts to accumulate. On the other hand, if you exercise rigorously and also your carb intake is low, you will have exhausted the glycogen very soon. But at the same time, you experience fatigue and tend to get dehydrated, which is not good for your health. Since there is little carbohydrate left and you carry on with the normal daily activities, you gradually get dehydrated. So, if you are opting for ketogenic diet, you ought to do away with rigorous exercise and intense weight training.

✓ **Hampered metabolism** - Since you are already dehydrated and you have lost muscles, your metabolism is completely hampered. This is indeed a cause of concern for the ones that are worried about muscle mass and muscle tone.

✓ **Risk of cancer** - If you are on low carbohydrate diet, and if you are not able to maintain it properly with the right amount of elements, you will have trouble with digestion and leads to bowel and constipation irregularities. This makes you susceptible to cardiovascular diseases and digestive cancer. Also, another cause of concern is that if you deprive yourself of legume, fruits, vegetables, and grains, it results in insufficient intake of potassium, vitamin C, and antioxidants. Also, intake of phytonutrients is compromised.

✓ **Subject to harmful ingredients** - Individuals on ketogenic diet tend to depend on sugar free chocolates, snack bars, and low carbohydrate ice creams and sandwiches. These artificial foods contain harmful ingredients like maltitol. Experts usually say that it is best to avoid artificial foods as these, especially if they are wrapped in tetra packs and packed with expiry dates.

✓ **Organs adversely affected** - Long term implications of low carbohydrate diet result in stress on major organs like kidneys and other organs.

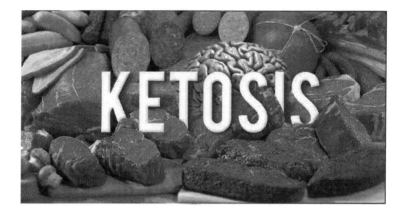

All about Ketosis

Ketosis can be referred to as a metabolic process, which is an ongoing process that th body regulates so that you can sustain all your activities well. When there is scarcity of carbohydrate from the food you take, the fat in your body is burnt to provide that energy, which your carbohydrate could not provide. As a consequence of the process, ketones are produced.

An important aspect that you must keep in mind is that you should not get confused between ketosis and ketoacidosis, which is an even more harmful procedure that takes place in the body. However, if you have adequate fat in your body, the ketones are not made use of.

Most importantly, a balanced diet is the best way to have a great metabolism as the optimum amount of fat is burnt and also whether the ketones will be burnt or not is regulated. And if a diabetic with untreated diabetes has ketosis, it is a sign that the hormone insulin is not being optimally utilized in the body.

However ketosis, over a period of time can become fatal as the chemical makeup of blood is altered. Also, it leads to dehydration, which can be life threatening. In fact, burning fat and utilizing ketones are 2 different metabolic pathways that occur in our body.

Research and extensive reveals that utilization of ketones is preferred over utilization of fat by the brain cells. This is because it has been proved that by utilizing ketones, there is 70% more release of energy for all the activities that individuals undertake.

How does ketosis work?

The liver breaks down fact, upon which fatty acid and glycerol is released. By the process of ketogenesis, fatty acid is broken down further. This results in the formation of acetoacetate, which is a ketone body. Two other types of ketone bodies are obtained known as BHB or Beta Hydroxybutyrate and Acetone. However, over the years, as you age, the number of ketone bodies released diminishes. An important aspect that you must keep in mind is that the body requires glucose for energy for the performance of different activities but carbohydrate is not required.

Another interesting factor is that excess protein is also converted into glucose in the blood stream. So, if you want optimum results from the ketogenic diet, it is essential that you maintain a high protein intake too along with high fat diet. This helps the liver to perform glucogenesis effectively.

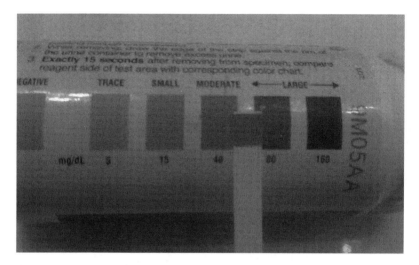

Why do we induce ketosis?

Ketosis has been found to be very effective in treating several disorders, the most common one being seizures. This therapy has been around since the 10920s. Inducing ketosis is helpful as it restricts or slows down the growth of certain types of cancers and cancerous tumors. It has been found to be 'correct' metabolic errors that take place, which essentially include obesity and diabetes.

Aside from this, certain degenerative conditions like Alzheimer's and Parkison's has also been treated efficiently by inducing ketosis.

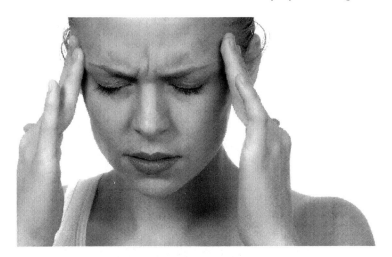

What are the symptoms of ketosis?

When it comes to symptoms, the duration for which these symptoms last usually differ from one individual to another. While in few it may last for a week, in few others, it may last for up to several days to weeks. The most pronounced symptoms include -

1.   Fatigue or feeling tired frequently

2.   Excessive thirst and most of the time

3.   Headache

4.   Fruity smell in breath and urine (ketosis breath)

5.   Dry mouth

6. Metallic taste on the rear side of the tongue

7. Disturbances in sleep

8. Weakness/lethargy

9. Dizziness

10. Abdominal pain

11. Nausea

12. Urinating frequently

13. Cold feet and hands

These symptoms may be an ongoing problem depending on how well or how long your body is taking to adapt to the ketogenic diet.

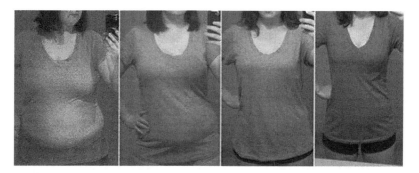

Ketogenic diet on weight loss

Obesity can be regarded as an epidemic that has spread across the length and breadth of the globe. It is one of the risk factors that can lead to metabolic disorders as well as a number of lifestyle disorders that include atherosclerosis, certain cancers, dyslipidemia, hypertension, and Type 2 diabetes. Also, it has come to the limelight after extensive studies that genetic predisposition alone is not responsible for these ailments. Carbohydrate intake along with lifestyle habits influence weight of an individual and consequently the BMI or the Body Mass Index.

One of the ways in which these lifestyle disorders can be tamed to a great extent is by nutritional intervention. It means changes in diet have to be brought about for optimum weight loss results. Ketogenic diet has been widely acclaimed and accepted by several individuals as one of the effective avenues of weight loss. Studies and experiments have shown that this form of diet has biochemical as well as physiological implications that contribute immensely to the effectiveness of the ketogenic diet.

According to clinicians and clinical studies, although KD or ketogenic diet is effective in treating epilepsy among children (KD has been found to be effective in the treatment of various other disorders like Alzheimer's, Parkinson's, Mitochondrial Disorder, Brain Tumor, Autism, Traumatic Brain Injury, ALS or Lou Gerhigs Disease), to name just a few, it has been found to be effective in weight loss too. It may be mentioned here that ketogenic diets inculcate in individuals a condition known as "physiological ketosis", which is markedly different from "pathological diabetic ketosis".

The effectiveness of the ketogenic diet can be attributed to the fact that the rate and quality of fat oxidation improves over time and is mirrored by RR or Respiratory Ratio, which decreases considerably. Although KD has been proved to be effective in weight loss, however, there are several debating issues regarding the mechanism that contributes to the same. While few experts are of the opinion that it works as there is suppression of appetite due to appetite controlling hormones or repletion of proteins, few others think that appetite is suppressed by the presence of ketone bodies.

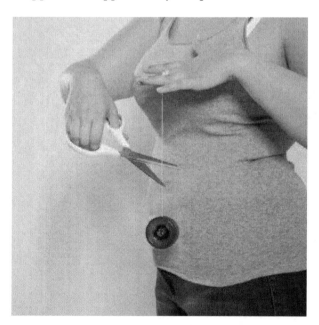

Yo-Yo effect of KD

Studies have implied that ketogenic diet helps in weight loss and yields better results as compared to low fat diets, at least on a short term basis. However, the nutritional intervention approach (KD effect) is regarded as successful depending on how much weight regain the individual undergoing ketogenic diet has recorded after a considerable period of time after taking the ketogenic diet. As such, few are of the opinion that the changes are "transient". This is known as the Yo-Yo effect or "weight cycling". As such how successfully you have been able to maintain your weight is one of the factors that will prove whether or not the nutritional approach has been successful or was able to attain the objective.

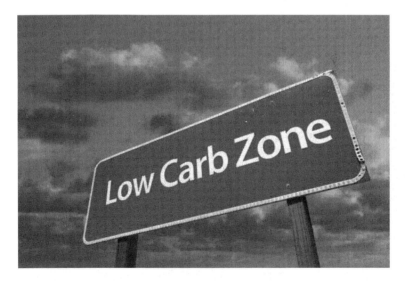

Ketogenic Diet versus Low Carb Diet

A diet that has less than 130gms or 150gms of carbohydrate as component is said to be a low carbohydrate diet. As far as ketogenic diets are concerned, these can be referred to as a kind of low carbohydrate diet plans, which is a part of the overall low carbohydrate diet. If you happen to consume carbohydrate, which is less than 50gms per day, you are said to be inducing a state of ketosis. This accounts for approximately 20gms to 30gms of net carbohydrate or it might be even less. Oftentimes, ketosis is confused with ketoacidosis, the latter being prevalent among the diabetics, the most. When ketosis results, ketone bodies are formed that provide the necessary energy for the daily activities instead of glucose, which is the case when ketosis does not occur.

You will come across many individuals that have over and over again enquired whether or not he is required to be in a state of ketosis in order to lose weight. However, experts are of the opinion that it is not always necessary to induce a state of ketosis in order to lose weight. If you consume a diet that comprises high fat, low carbohydrate, and adequate protein, it makes you less hungry. As such, you tend to feel full most of the time and your appetite diminishes. This can help you to consume less food.

Chapter 2

DIGGING DEEPER

Defining net carbs

The principle on which net carbs is based encompasses the fact that not all carbohydrates impact the body in a similar manner. The carbohydrates that have high glycemic index are the ones that are refined/simple starches as well as sugars. It means that these food items that have higher glycemic index tend to raise your blood sugar level quickly just after you have consumed these food items. The simple sugars occurring in excess are usually stored as fat in the body. White rice, sweetmeat, white bread, and potatoes are classical examples of this type of carbohydrate.

There are yet other types of carbohydrates found in fruits, vegetables, and whole grain the movement of which is slow as they pass through the digestive system. Majority of these carbohydrates do not get digested easily or at all.

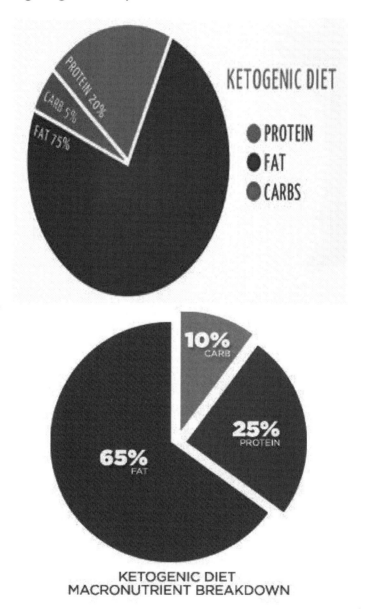

KETOGENIC DIET
MACRONUTRIENT BREAKDOWN

When it comes to explaining the meaning of net carb, it is the carbohydrate that is "accepted by your body as carbohydrate. For these reasons, the nutritional facts that are mentioned on the labels of food products are important as they carry the information about the nutritional value of each ingredient that has been used in the food item.

In order to calculate the net carb, you have to calculate the total carbohydrate present in any food item and then subtract the percentage or amount of fiber and alcohol that is also present in the food item. You will have to subtract the fiber and alcohol amount because these 2 ingredients do not contribute to raising your blood sugar levels. And they impact the blood sugar level in the minimum possible way.

Importance of eliminating dairy products

It is a well known fact that the objective of weight loss is to get rid of as much fat tissue as possible; it has been observed that to some extent there is loss of lean tissue as well. However, experts are of the opinion that loss of lean tissue has been held responsible for weight regain despite the fact that during any weight loss program, individuals undergoing the training adhere religiously to exercise regime and maintain dietary restrictions.

Earlier studies have also revealed that calcium helps in facilitating and promoting breakdown of fat cells, thereby helping in weight loss. According to Rachel Novotny, Chair and professor in the department of human nutrition, food, and animal sciences, University of Hawaii, dairy has greater impact on fat loss especially trunk fat as compared to calcium alone.

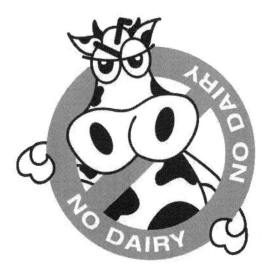

The weight loss effect of dairy can be primarily attributed to the calcium content present in dairy. This can be safely said because according to Novotny, minerals present in the dairy like magnesium and phosphorus can foster breakdown of fat brought about by calcium within the cells. Similarly, the protein content that is present in the dairy help in retaining muscles and catalyzes metabolism in a positive manner, thereby making weight loss effective by dairy consumption.

Studies conducted by Josse et al, have shown how calcium and protein impact weight loss in obese and overweight people. Reports from the study suggest that consumption of high dairy food items as well as high protein food items was found to be effective in facilitating retention of lean muscle mass as well as burning fat.

It goes without saying that you ought to incorporate dairy products in your diet, which might include yogurt, cheese, and milk. Aside from being reliable source of vitamins, zinc, and protein, it has been observed that dairy products are a good source of calcium. Research has shown that dairy products help in weight loss. For instance, studies have proved that children that drink milk have lower body mass. Also, individuals that drink milk and consume dairy products tend to be slimmer.

Although consuming cheese, yogurt, and milk are good for deriving the essential nutrients, yet there are several alternatives of milk and dairy products that can help in weight loss. These include semi skimmed as well as skimmed milk, cheese with low fat content, and low fat yogurts. It has been found that low fat skimmed milk (a pint) has 190 calories or 0.6gms of fat.

An important aspect that you ought to remember is that consuming low fat dairy products does not necessarily mean that you will have less of the essential nutrients. In fact, if you consume low fat dairy, it can help in weight loss. If you are on ketogenic diet, the best thing you can do about dairy products is that make sure you consume dairy products in moderation. If you are not lactose intolerant, you can carry on with your dairy portions but in moderation. So, you don't have to give up your favorite ice cream, yogurt, or cheese.

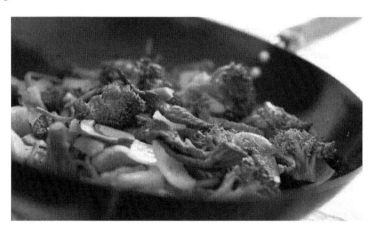

Effect of fiber on carbohydrate absorption

Fiber is also included among carbohydrates, similar to starch and sugars, however, as the human body does not break down the fiber, it does not contribute to the intake of calorie that is the case with other carbohydrates. We know that the impact of carbohydrate on blood glucose level is high. So, what is the impact of fiber on carbohydrate absorption? Let us see. As mentioned above, fiber does not raise blood glucose level because it is not digested. As such, fiber is recommended for the ones suffering from diabetes. However, there are other food items that aside from containing fiber also contain non-fiber carbohydrate. These essentially include the likes of pastas, fruits, vegetables, cereals, and whole grain breads. These also contain sugar and starch. So, when you decide to incorporate fiber in your weight loss regime or any meal plan that you are embarking upon, you have to take these non fiber carbohydrate content into account and select the appropriate type of fiber (insoluble).

As per a report that was furnished upon conducting a study and was published in New England Journal of Medicine, indicated that diabetics that consumed approximately 50gms of fiber daily were in a better position to control their blood sugar levels. Ideally, it is said that at least 20gms to 25gms of fiber should be consumed every day.

There are 2 types of fibers, namely, soluble as well as insoluble fiber. An example of insoluble fiber is whole wheat bran. These fibers are known to aid in the health of your digestive tract. On the other hand, soluble fibers aid in lowering levels of cholesterol and aids in maintaining proper blood glucose level. A typical example of this type of fiber is oatmeal.

Since the body is not able to digest fiber, it plays a crucial role in digestion. Soluble fibers as mentioned above (a few more example include beans, blueberries, nuts, and cucumbers) dissolve to give a gel-like consistency, which slows down digestion. This is one reason why you feel full after eating few food items. This particular property of fiber and its impact on digestion has been found to be effective in the control of weight. This principle works when you try to incorporate carbohydrate and fiber in your weight loss regime. You will come across many types of foods that contain both types of fibers- soluble as well as insoluble.

According to a write up that was published in "Journal of the American College of Nutrition", way back in the year 2009, there are some food items like white kidney beans that comprise substances that aid in preventing the absorption of carbohydrate. This is usually done by acting on the enzymes that break down the carbohydrates. The enzyme amylase present in saliva initiates the process of carbohydrate digestion. However, it has also been observed that an individual would not possibly get adequate substances that can prevent amylase from working on carbohydrate just by consuming foods alone, as such; supplements are required to help amylase work in a manner that will prohibit or limit the absorption of carbohydrate.

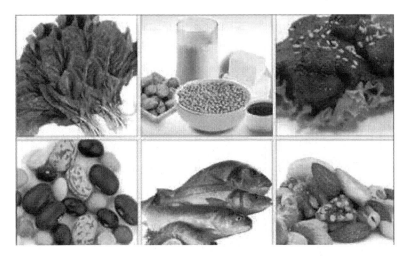

Fiber weight loss vs. fullness

If you have embarked upon a journey of weight loss, you will have to adopt all measures that prevent you from binge eating all the wrong types of foods. There are many ways in which you can help yourself to lose weight and lead a healthy life. These days, we find that obesity, hypertension, cardiac diseases, certain types of cancer, gall bladder diseases, and other ailments are all consequences of sedentary lifestyle, and inappropriate methods of food intake. How will fiber aid in weight loss? And how will "feeling full" aid in weight loss? Let us find out.

More and more people are turning to what is known as "energy density" weight loss. Just as consuming high fat foods and low carb foods help in weight loss in ketogenic diet has been found to be effective, inducing the feeling of fullness and incorporating fiber in your daily diet intake also yields results in weight loss. Let us see how both these concepts help you in weight loss.

Energy density can be referred to as the number of calories that a particular food contains. It basically means the number of calories present in any food. So, how will the concept of energy density aid weight loss? A food that is regarded as high density usually has a higher number of calories in a comparatively less amount of food. On the other hand, low energy density means fewer calories in large amount of food. When you are aiming at weight loss, it is best to take low energy density food. In other words, your goal will be to eat more food that contains least calories. This is a trick that most of the dieting individuals opt for because it makes them feel fuller. What makes a food of higher energy density or lower energy density? There are many **factors that contribute to density of foods**, namely,

✓ **Fiber** - Foods that are rich in fiber offer greater volume. Also, they take longer to get digested, one of the main reasons that make you feel full and for a long spell. So, you are consuming lesser calories by eating more volume of food. Classical example of this type of fiber is popcorn. It is larger in volume but has fewer calories.

✓ **Water** - Another factor that contributes to the volume of food is water. You can consume enough fruits and vegetables that have higher water content. And they do not have very high calories. However, you have to select those types of foods that satisfy the criteria of contributing to higher volume of food.

Aside from water and fiber, fat also contributes to higher volume in any food item.

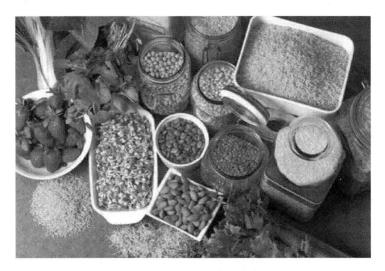

Type of fiber that contributes to fullness is insoluble fiber. There are 2 categories of fiber, namely, soluble and insoluble. While soluble fiber dissolves and is easily digested, it does not make you feel full.

Instead, it regulates blood glucose level. However, insoluble fiber is not easily digested and collects water as it moves through the intestine slowly providing the sense of fullness.

The rule of the thumb is that if you are able to take advantage of the property of the insoluble fiber, you will feel full for a longer time. Also, your appetite will be regulated accordingly. So, dieticians or clinicians directing patients for weight loss recommend increased consumption of fiber in the diet, which makes you feel full for a longer time. It has also been observed that aside from the fiber content, if you take time and chew your food, it produces more saliva as well as juices in the stomach that aid digestion.

The secret to healthy living and food habit is not skipping your breakfast. The ones that have managed to shed weight and not let it come back again (no weight regain) eat breakfast on a regular basis. This fact was provided by the National Weight Control Registry. And the main food that kept the weight off in these individuals is cereal.

Chapter 3

DOING IT THE RIGHT WAY

Let's get started!

Starting a ketogenic diet will take some time to show results as your body starts to acclimatize to the new metabolism pathway. Generally speaking, the effects should start showing anytime between 2 weeks and 4 weeks. The main objective of a ketogenic diet is to achieve a state, which is referred to as ketosis. This is a simple metabolic process in which the body burns out fat from the body and provides energy not from glucose but from ketones. This state is said to be favorable for individuals at those times when your body does not have enough energy to support your daily activities.

There are many people that confuse ketosis with ketoacidosis, which is a critical state and should be prevented by all means as it can have threatening consequences. The rule of thumb in a ketogenic diet is to have a diet that is low in carbohydrate. However, an important aspect that you must remember is that not all low carbohydrate diets are essentially ketogenic. But remember that not all low carbohydrate diets are ketogenic diets. The main difference between a ketogenic diet and a low carbohydrate diet is the amount of protein and fat that you can be allowed to consume every day.

Prior to starting this diet, there are few questions that you have to find answers to. These are crucial as they might impact your health. So, ask the following questions first-

✓ Are you eligible to opt for the ketogenic diet? If it is 'yes', you can go ahead and if it is 'no',

✓ Who cannot opt for this diet and why? Know the medical contraindications thoroughly,

✓ Are there side effects of the diet?

✓ Benefits of the diet

✓ Drawbacks of the diet

✓ Do the benefits surpass the drawbacks?

✓ If you have pre-existing medical conditions like you suffer from kidney and heart ailments, are you eligible?

✓ If you are breastfeeding and pregnant, can you opt for the diet?

These are just few of the questions that you can ask your GP. But it is always better in the interest of your health to know what you can expect and get the facts straight.

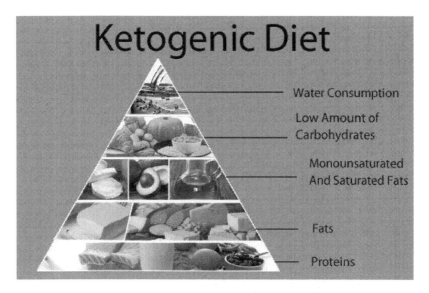

The step wise approach to a ketogenic diet has been listed below-

✓ Once you are confident about the questions above and you are eligible for the same, take into account the amount of carbohydrate, fat, and protein that you will be allowed to consume.

✓ The amount of carbohydrate, fat, and protein you take will essentially depend on the height, body weight, exercise, and gender of the individual undertaking the diet.

✓ The ketogenic diet requires you to monitor closely the carbohydrate you take daily. The consumption should be between 20gms/day and 60gms/day.

✓ As far as protein is concerned, it has to be moderate. As mentioned above, it will depend upon the gender, height, exercise, and weight.

✓ You will have to incorporate fat content too.

✓ An important aspect is that the ratios of the individual elements (fat, protein, carbohydrate, and exercise regime) will ensure whether or not you will be able to stay in ketosis even after you have continued with the diet for quite some time. This is because unless the ratios between the elements are right, many individuals have regained their weight again.

✓ Ideally, you have to derive 70% to 75% calories from fat, 5% to 10% from carbohydrates, and 20% to 25% from protein. This is the daily bifurcation of the elements that you have to adhere to.

✓ It may be mentioned here that although the amount of fat you consume daily does not impact blood glucose level but the amount of protein you consume daily will impact the blood insulin level. So, if you take higher protein amount daily, it will drive up the level of blood insulin. As a result the substrate for ketosis will not be formed as the body's ability to burn fat will be hampered. As such, the amount of protein you take is crucial to the success of a ketogenic diet.

✓ Be prepared to count fat, carbohydrate, and protein intake.

✓ Decide upon the meals (main dishes as well as side dishes and dessert, soups and salads).

✓ Avoid junk and fast foods and the ones that you are not supposed to eat.

✓ Hydration is important. Try to stay as much hydrated as possible.

✓ Stay away from foods that have high carbohydrate content.

✓ And last but not the least stay motivated.

✓ Monitor the results closely.

✓ Remember diet alone may not give you the desired results, so you will be required to exercise too.

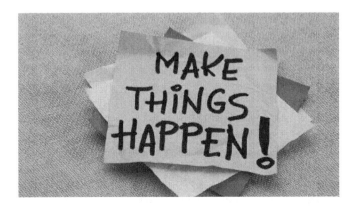

Trick to staying motivated

It goes without saying that ketogenic diet is undoubtedly good for your health. But oftentimes, it has come to light that most of the people left the diet plan midway and were not able to take the entire course of the diet to completion. As such, it is of utmost importance to stay motivated at all times. You can do the following to stay motivated at all times. Take a look-

✓ **Gather support** - One of the best ways to stay motivated is to get support from the ones that are also undergoing the same diet plan. If you talk to them, understand how they are able to sustain the diet, you will feel much better. Alternatively, you will find many online forums where detailed discussions take place related to different topics. So, you can visit one such forum that deals with ketogenic diet and stay motivated by drawing inspiration from them.

✓ **Avoid negative feedback** - If you find people saying the adverse about the outcome of the ketogenic diet, stay away from such criticism. Instead, just focus on what you have opted for. Remember, the metabolic rate always differs from one person to another. So, the results might as well differ. So, if someone approaches you and insists that you stop the diet plan as it will not yield results, do not pay heed to these talks.

✓ **Don't let deviation disappoint you** - If at any point of time, you have eaten some food item that you are not supposed to eat, don't feel guilty. Getting into a ketogenic diet plan is after all a lifestyle change and you might take some time to streamline the diet plan. Give yourself time, don't rush, and try to adhere to the diet religiously at all times. But don't keep any stones unturned in following the diet plan. But it does not mean that every time you get out of the diet and feel bad about it and start it again. This is because when you start the diet, remember, it takes time to get into a state of ketosis. So, if you happen to get out of ketosis again, you will have to regain the state of ketosis again. So, keep this mind that you will be playing and jeopardizing the rate of metabolism if you get out and get in again and again in the state of ketosis.

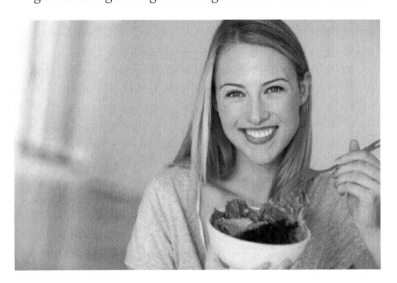

Eating right-secret to success

With more time being spent at the desk, less of exercise, more of harmful calorie intake, sedentary lifestyle, cut throat competition, striving hard to survive competition at workplace, more and more people are subjecting themselves to stress. Life is full of ups and downs and in an effort to religiously follow Darwin's concept of "Survival of the fittest", our life oftentimes falls like a pack of cards as we tend to play our cards wrong!

Yes, we tend to get so much involved in our mundane life; we forget that we can increase our lifespan by leading a healthy lifestyle. Thankfully, we can "turn back the clock" and to some extent reverse the damage we have inflicted on ourselves. One of the best ways to do so is follow a healthy diet and stay healthy. However, losing weight does not necessarily mean that you lose weight only to regain it after a couple of weeks. You have to attain that "dream weight" and stay there as long as you can. It can be challenging, nevertheless, it is not impossible. So, gear up for a healthy life!

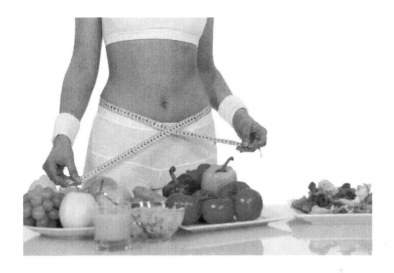

Using healthy foods as weapons to lose weight - Planning well is the mantra of success when it comes to eating right and staying fit. It is best to avoid foods that harm us. But despite knowing that a particular group of food might harm us, we tend to overlook the negative aspects of the food because we relish the taste of it. But exercising self restraint is another mantra of success and rule of thumb, when it comes to choosing the right kind of food for staying healthy.

When you decided to eat healthy, plan out your food intake, the main dishes, the side dishes, snacks, soups, and desserts so that you can measure the calories you are taking and not consuming harmful calories. In the following paragraphs, we will see how you can stay healthy and eat right.

✓ **Eat fat to tame fat** - While saturated fats found in processed foods (meat, crackers, and cookies) are harmful for you, there are unsaturated fats and if you consume a diet that is rich in the right kind of fat can be good for your waist diameter. Monosaturated fatty acids also known as MUFAs are found in olive oil, avocados, and nuts and are found to be effective in reducing fat in the belly area. Polyunsaturated fatty acids also known as PUFAs are also good and found in fish and the oil from fish. Studies have proved that consuming PUFA will enhance the rate of metabolism even when you are in a resting mode. If you consume the right kind of fat, it will also make you feel full. As a result, your appetite will be controlled and you won't munch on unhealthy snacks.

✓ **Dairy products reduce fat** - Dairy products help in weight loss. We have discussed about the role of dairy in weight loss in the preceding paragraphs. Studies have revealed that individuals with calcium deficiency have fat mass. Also, yogurt, milk, cheese (non fat), which are "dairy sources of calcium" are effective in weight loss. Ideally, if you take 3 dairy servings on a daily basis, you will find a marked difference in your weight.

✓ **Chocolate helps in weight loss** - Consume those chocolates that have a higher cocoa content and less of sugar. Studies conducted on mice revealed that consuming cocoa, which is rich in antioxidants, the lifespan of these animals improved. As it is said that flavonoid improves mood and was found to have an antiaging effect on the mice. The study was conducted to conform whether or not in obese diabetic mice the lifespan could be improved. It was found that consuming a certain amount of cocoa delayed degeneration of aortic arteries and also had a positive impact on fat deposition.

✓ **Couple up right diet with right amount of exercise** - If you think that you can eat all those harmful calories as you are exercising rigorously daily, you are wrong. It has been proved through experiments and studies that exercise alone could impact only about 3% of the total weight loss regime, the rest has to be attributed by the right kind of food intake.

✓ **Interval training versus cardio sessions** - While few are of the opinion that cardio sessions can yield better results, there are yet few individuals that believe that interval training can be more effective in weight loss. Aside from the right form of exercise, taking the right kind of food also had a positive impact on your health.

✓ **Hydration** - Drink water to your heart's content. This is a universal solvent and one of the best forms of liquid that can keep you cool, keep your entire system healthy, and keep you away from several kinds of ailments. Also, it is seen that prior to the major meals if you drink a specific amount of water, you tend to eat less at the table. Alternatively, if you are not content with just water, you can also drink beverages that are devoid of sugar.

✓ **Avoid mindless eating** - Snacking time can be a challenging time for all of us. The type of snacks we eat matters most especially at night time. We generally tend to gulp down chips mindlessly if we are sitting in front of the television and watching our favorite programs. Close the kitchen when you retire to bed or if you are sitting down to watch TV. Also, keep those harmful snacks locked inside the kitchen when you sit to watch TV.

✓ **Don't deprive yourself of your favorite food** - You might be under the impression that trying to lose weight means you have to stop all your favorite foods altogether. But this is not true. Staying away from the food items you love but ones that are rich in fat will only compel you to reach out for them. So, instead of eating these snacks as you used to, minimize the intake. For instance, earlier if you used to buy 2 packets of that snacks, now buy just half or one.

✓ **Spread food intake over the day** - It goes without saying that if th food intake is less than what you burn, your weight loss regime will be effective. In other words, if the number of calories you are consuming is less as compared to the calories you are burning; your weight loss program will work best. You can have several "mini meals" throughout the day. And when you do so, the most number of mini meals should be planned during the day. As evening approaches, you should reduce intake of calories and dinner should be last, which should never be very heavy. Have a light dinner.

✓ **Retire to bed in time** - Ever since we went to school, we were told "early to bed early to rise, makes you healthy, wealthy, and wise". In fact, this is true. If you have dinner at 7.30Pm, give yourself sometime and retire to bed 3 hours after you have had your dinner. This helps in metabolism and you tend to lose weight early. Also, the carbohydrate intake for dinner should be minimal.

✓ **Protein is important** - Regardless of the number of mini meals you are eating, incorporate protein in every meal. It gives you a "fill up" feeling and preserves your muscles. Also it helps in burning fat. Ideal examples of protein that you can incorporate in your diet include lean meat, egg whites, seafood, soy, beans, nuts, yogurt, and cheese.

✓ **Taste matters** - It has been observed that if you can have a meal that is tasty with spices and chilies, you have a much more fulfilling meal.

✓ **Preserve healthy foods** - One of the main concerns of weight regain is that we tend to binge eat especially when it comes to snacking. As such, you can stuff your refrigerator with healthy foods like canned tomatoes, salad greens, fat reduced cheese, pasta made of whole grain, vegetables (frozen), chicken breast, and tortillas.

✓ **Eating out - Plan your portion** - If you plan to eat out at a food joint or restaurant, order for food that is the same as baby portion. In this way you will not overeat and at the same time you will be able to control your food intake and consequently calorie intake too.

✓ **Swap healthy foods** - If you used to eat snacks that included burger and high calorie cookies, swap these unhealthy foods with vegetables. Instead of burgers and pasta, have a cup of boiled vegetables with some flavor added to it. According to Cynthia Sass, spokeswoman for American Dietetic Association, "You can save from 100-200 calories if you reduce the portion of starch on your plate and increase the amount of vegetables".

✓ **Don't skip breakfast** - It has been observed that if you skip breakfast, you tend to feel hungrier later during the day, which leads to eating even more. And when you feel hungry when you are working at your workstation, the thought process works in a different manner. You become complacent with the healthy foods and think that eating unhealthy food just once will not harm your body. Nevertheless, this habit of binging harms even more and the calorie intake throughout the day becomes haywire.

✓ **Fiber is important** - Consuming fiber has a number of benefits. It helps in digestion, controls cholesterol, makes bowel movements smooth, and most importantly aids in weight loss. Ideally, it is recommended that 25gms of fiber ought to be included in daily diet. While this figure holds true in the case of women for men, it is 38gms. Add whole grain foods, beans, oatmeal, vegetables, and fruits to your daily diet. Space out the consumption accordingly.

✓ **Opt for steady weight loss** - Experts are of the opinion that if you lose weight abruptly, it is harmful. Instead, you should lose weight steadily and not rush into weight losing spree. After all, you cannot play havoc with your metabolism. It will affect you adversely.

✓ **Add more vegetables and fruits to your diet** - Fruits and vegetables are filling and will not make you feel hungry easily. Have as much fruits and vegetables as you can on a daily basis.

Aside from the tips for healthy eating mentioned above, other things that you can do to keep tab on your weight is to weigh weekly or may be twice a week. Enjoy life and stay healthy.

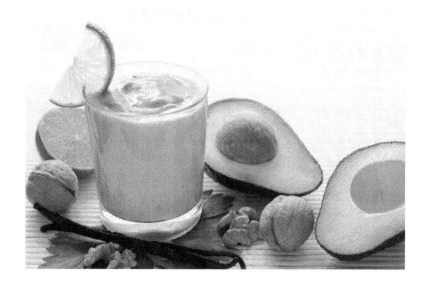

Food & drinks that Keto pros approve of

When you have started living on a ketogenic diet and if you are still new to the concept, you might have confusion before you pop just about anything in your mouth. But this list of foods will help you to decide what you should reach out for and what you should avoid. The list has been prepared in such a manner that will help you to decide the foods that you can take on a regular basis, the ones that can be taken occasionally, and the ones that you ought to avoid completely. So, check out the list first and jumpstart on your ketogenic diet right away!

Given below is a list of food items and beverages that you can consume without any inhibitions. These are as follows-

Eat regularly

- ✓ Swiss chard
- ✓ Bamboo shoots
- ✓ Bok choy
- ✓ Radicchio
- ✓ Chives
- ✓ Lettuce
- ✓ Chard
- ✓ Spinach
- ✓ Asparagus
- ✓ Zucchini
- ✓ Spaghetti squash
- ✓ Summer squash

- ✓ Cucumber

- ✓ Celery stalk

- ✓ Kale

- ✓ Radishes

- ✓ kohlrabi

You can eat the above non starchy vegetables.

- ✓ Avocado

- ✓ Macadamia nuts

- ✓ Coconut

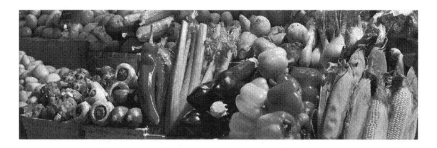

As far as fruits, seeds, and nuts are concerned, your options are mentioned above.

- ✓ Goat

✓ Venison

✓ Lamb

✓ Beef

✓ Poultry

✓ Pastured pork

✓ Gelatin

✓ Heart

✓ Organ meats

✓ Liver

✓ Kidneys

✓ Offal

✓ Butter

✓ Ghee

✓ Eggs

Animal sources mentioned above can be ideal for ketogenic diet.

✓ Olive oil (Monosaturated)

✓ Saturated fat - coconut oil, butter, ghee, goose fat, tallow, chicken fat, clarified butter, and duck fat

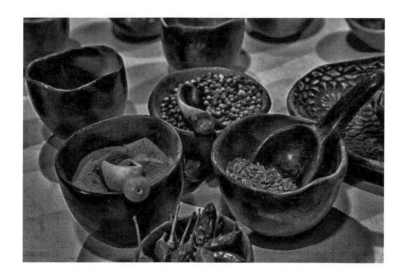

Beverages and spices/condiments

✓   Still water

✓   Black coffee with cream

✓   Coconut milk

✓   Tea (herbal as well as black)

✓   Cracklings of pork rinds

✓   Pesto

✓   Mustard

✓   Mayonnaise

✓   Bone broth

✓   Whey protein

✓ Egg white lecithin

✓ Zest

✓ Lime juice

✓ Lemon

✓ Herbs

✓ Spices

Avoid artificial sweeteners and additives

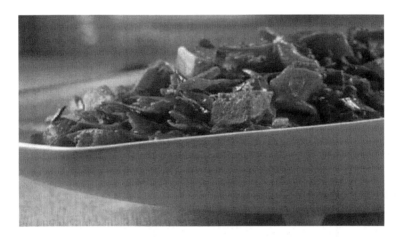

Ideal for occasional consumption

The list of food items that are mentioned below can be consumed

once in a while but not on a regular basis. These essentially include-

✓ Red cabbage

✓ Turnip

- ✓ White cabbage
- ✓ Broccoli
- ✓ Cauliflower
- ✓ Fennel
- ✓ Rutabaga
- ✓ Brussels sprouts
- ✓ Parsley root
- ✓ Eggplant
- ✓ Pepper
- ✓ Tomatoes
- ✓ Onion
- ✓ Garlic
- ✓ Winter squash
- ✓ Spring onion
- ✓ Leek
- ✓ Mushrooms
- ✓ Bean sprouts
- ✓ Sugar snap peas
- ✓ French artichokes
- ✓ Wax beans

- ✓ Water chestnuts

- ✓ Blueberries

- ✓ Raspberries

- ✓ Cranberries

- ✓ Blackberries

- ✓ Olives

- ✓ Rhubarb

- ✓ Strawberries

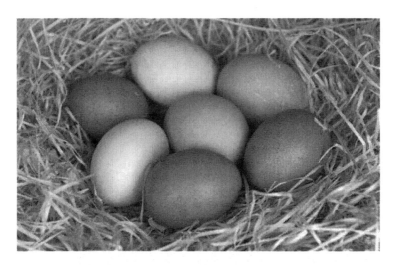

The above food items fall in the category of **fruits, mushroom, and vegetables**.

- ✓ Ghee

- ✓ Eggs

✓   Poultry

✓   Beef

✓   Plain yogurt

✓   Cottage cheese

✓   Sour cream

✓   Cheese

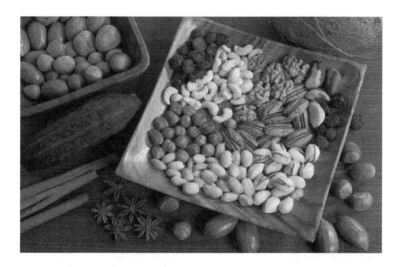

It is best not to eat farmed pork as the concentration of Omega 6 is very high. Also, it is better not to eat foods that are labeled as "low fat". When you eat bacon, make sure you don't eat the ones that have added starch as well as preservatives. If your intake of antioxidants is quite high, you can afford to take some preservatives that have nitrate as one of the ingredients.

✓   Almonds

- ✓ Pecans

- ✓ Hazelnuts

- ✓ Flaxseed

- ✓ Pumpkin seeds

- ✓ Walnuts

- ✓ Pine nuts

- ✓ Sunflower seeds

- ✓ Hemp seeds

- ✓ Sesame seeds

- ✓ Brazil nuts (you can consume Brazil nuts occasionally as they have a high content of selenium)

- ✓ Celery root

- ✓ Sweet potato

- ✓ Beetroot

- ✓ Parsnip

- ✓ Carrot

- ✓ Watermelon

- ✓ Apricot

- ✓ Nectarine

- ✓ Kiwifruit

✓ Plums

✓ Figs

✓ Ears

✓ Grapefruit

✓ Peach

✓ Apple

✓ Raisins

✓ Dates

✓ Chestnuts

✓ Dragon fruit

✓ Honeydew melons

✓ Cashew nuts

✓ Pistachios

Raisins and dates should be eaten occasionally only.

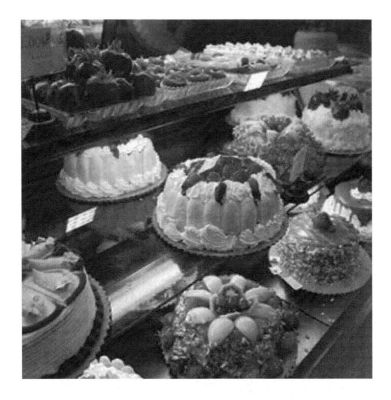

Foods that you should **avoid completely** include the following-

✓ Sugary drinks

✓ Sugar

✓ Fish and pork (factory farmed)

✓ Products that contain gluten

✓ Grains

✓ Trans fat

✓ Excessive omega 6

✓   Processed oils

✓   Legumes

✓   White potatoes

✓   Artificial sweeteners

✓   Monosodium glutamate

✓   Additives

✓   Colorings

✓   Preservatives

✓   BPAs

✓   Any product that is labeled "low carb", "low fat", and "low calorie".

The best way to incorporate all the healthy food items (the ones that you can eat while on ketogenic diet) is to include them in your diet plan and add them one at a time as and when your dietician will recommend or suggest.

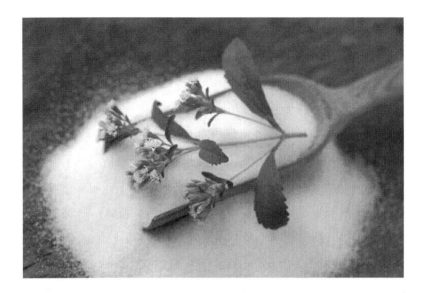

Pick the right spices & sweeteners

Spices and sweeteners are also to be taken in moderation or there are few brands of sweeteners that have to be avoided completely. Given below are the spices and condiments that can be taken occasionally and the ones that have to be avoided completely. Check the list.

✓ Sugar free chewing gums as well as mints can be taken occasionally

✓ Soy lecithin is to be avoided

✓ Tomato products that are sugar free like puree, ketchup, and passata can be taken occasionally.

✓ You can take carob powder and cocoa at times

✓ Healthy sweeteners like Erythritol, Stevia, and Swerve can be taken at times

✓ You can also take thickeners like xanthum gum and arrowroot powder from time to time.

✓ If you are sensitive to gluten, then you have to avoid Tamari soy sauce

✓ Mustard

✓ Salsas

✓ Capers

✓ Mayonnaise

✓ Tabasco

✓ Cider and wine vinegars

✓ Horseradish

✓ Sugar free pickles

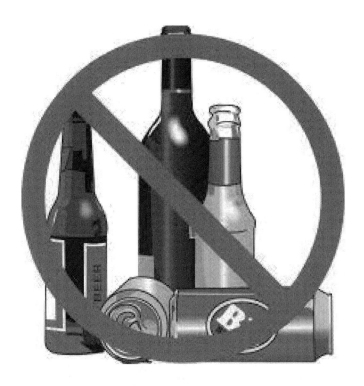

What about alcohol?

It goes without saying that while you are on a ketogenic diet, if you have to party, it becomes difficult to decide what you should have and what you shouldn't. This holds true especially for the alcohol or liquor. An important aspect that you have to keep in mind is that hard liquor is made up of ingredients that are by themselves full of calories like grains, sugar, fruits, and potatoes. However, when the distillation as well as fermentation process takes place the sugar content in the hard liquor gets converted into ethyl alcohol. Although there are many that believe that it is best to take light beer and dry wine as they are devoid of carbohydrates. However, this is not the case.

Generally speaking, there is content of 7gm to 20gm net carbohydrates in light beer and dry wine. So, if anyone has misguided you saying that these two drinks do not contain carbohydrate, he is misleading you. So, be well informed. Experts are of the opinion that it is best not to drink any kind of liquor especially when you are on ketogenic diet and trying to lose weight.

Studies have revealed that excessive consumption of alcohol while on ketogenic diet usually inhibits the fat burning process. So, when you are drinking the following, namely, beer, cocktails, flavored liquor, wine, syrups, juice, and soda, make sure you do so in moderation or not consume at all as these contain carbohydrates for which you might lose weight a little late.

It is alright to drink the following while you are on ketogenic diet but remember, all these drinks contain high amount of calories and is not recommended for weight loss as the process gets delayed if consumed on a regular basis.

✓ **Whisky** - Corn, wheat, barley, fermented grain, and rye make up whisky. This drink comprises alcohol in the percentage between 35 and 50. Since this drink is devoid of carbohydrates, it is regarded as a safe drink while you are on a ketogenic diet. Two variation of this category of drink include Scotch whisky and bourbon.

✓ **Vodka** - The volume of alcohol in this drink varies between 35% and 50% and is made up of rye, wheat, and potatoes. Opt for Vodka that does not have any flavor. And if at all you opt for flavored Vodka, buy the ones that have zero carbohydrate. This is because few varieties of Vodka also contain syrup and sugar.

✓ **Tequila** - The volume of alcohol in Tequila is only 40%. It is made up of agave plant. The taste of this drink will differ depending on its place of origin. You don't have to worry about choosing any variation of this drink and there is not too many flavored variety of the same.

✓ **Gin** - Made of grain base and with a volume of alcohol of 35%, the main ingredients of the drink is lime/lemon/orange. Avoid Sloe gin as these are made up of sugars and syrup and have added carbohydrates in them.

✓ **Rum** - Rum is from sugarcane/molasses. It is available in a variety of flavors. This drink is zero carb and zero carbohydrate too. However, stay away from the ones that are flavored. The volume of alcohol is 35%.

It has been observed that if you drink alcohol, your state of ketosis will be strengthened further. However, this holds true if you are having hard liquor. The more you drink alcohol, the more ketones your liver metabolizes. Also, consumed alcohol gets converted into triglycerides, which positively impacts ketone production. However, a condition known as alcohol ketoacidosis should be avoided at all cost. This condition occurs when people have consumed large volumes of alcohol without having any solid food.

Chapter 4

KETO FOOD & DIET THERAPY

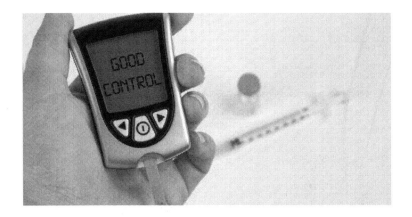

Controlling blood sugar with Keto diet

S tudies have proved that the ketogenic diet has the capacity to control blood glucose levels. In fact, it tends to decrease the blood glucose level in individuals that suffer from Type 2 diabetes. This is because it has been observed that consumption of carbohydrates tend to get converted into blood sugar that raises the blood glucose level in the blood. As such, if you are already diabetic, you have to control your carbohydrate intake.

Since ketogenic diet comprises intake of low carbohydrate, your intake of carbohydrate also gets reduced, which in turn helps in controlling blood glucose level. However, in the ketogenic diet, you derive energy from fat and not from glucose as there is a state called ketosis that you have to achieve.

In case of non diabetic individuals, this should not be a matter of concern, but in case of diabetics, attaining a state of ketosis can sometimes be dangerous. This is because having ketones in excess can lead to a dangerous state called DKA or diabetic ketoacidosis.

Diabetes ketoacidosis is mostly found in individuals suffering from Type 1 diabetes. Nevertheless, this state of raised ketones in the blood cannot be ruled out in people with Type 2 diabetes too. According to the American Diabetes Association, it is best to get your blood sugar tested for DKA especially if your blood sugar level is higher than 240mg/dl.

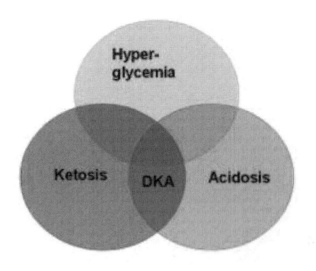

You are suffering from diabetes ketoacidosis if you complain of the following symptoms-

✓ Dry mouth

✓ Nausea

✓ Frequent urination

✓ Fruit like smell in your breath

✓ Uncontrolled blood sugar

✓ Breathing problem

There is a difference between a low carbohydrate diet and a ketogenic diet and this is in terms of carbohydrate intake primarily. As such, it needs monitoring on a regular basis. In individuals with type 1 and type 2 diabetes if ketogenic diet is being recommended, it is essential that the blood glucose level and level of ketones in the blood has to be monitored regularly in order to keep a check so that no adverse effects occur.

In a nut shell, ketogenic diet is ideal for diabetics with Type 2 diabetes as the symptoms can be controlled to a great extent. Also, patients with Type 2 diabetes will complain of lesser symptoms related to diabetes and may also have to depend less on medicines.

Most importantly, the results differ from one person to another. This is because while few individuals will adhere to the restriction religiously, there will be few that will opt out of the diet midway as they find it difficult to follow the restrictions well. So, experts are of the opinion that if you are not sure of continuing with the diet, it is best not to embark upon the same. Only if you think that you can confidently complete the ketogenic diet regime, should you start with the diet.

Prior to starting the diet, it is best to talk to your doctor first and if he thinks that you are eligible for the diet, you can start it promptly and enjoy the benefits of the same.

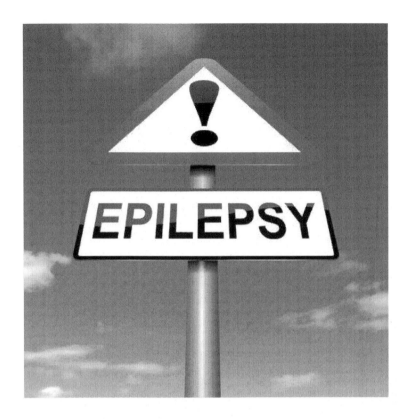

Keto therapy for epilepsy

According to statistical data, in the United is States alone, the average incidence is 150,000. In other words, it can be safely said that 49 out of 100,000 individuals will develop epilepsy annually. The typical age group that is susceptible to epilepsy seizures is in elderly people and children. The number of people with epilepsy ranges between 1.3 million and 2.8 million.

The ketogenic diet comprises high intake of fat, low carbohydrate, and low protein. This diet is recommended by doctors to treat children suffering from severe bouts of epilepsy and the ones that medicines have failed to heal. The diet is high in fat content and is taken in form of fatty foods that include cream, oil, margarine, and butter. Also, the keto diet has adequate protein for your child and small quantity of carbohydrate.

Prior to starting the diet for epilepsy, you have to keep in mind that this diet is totally different as compared to what other children have and are used to eating. There are restrictions that need to be followed in this diet. So, it requires a lot of effort in maintaining the same.

Studies reveal that in 1/3 of epilepsy affected children when subjected to ketogenic diet yield positive results and that 90% of them have shown marked improvement in seizures. At least, 50% of the children have reduced incidence of seizures, while there are many that discontinue the diet as they fail to adhere to the restrictions and find it difficult to pursue further treatment of epilepsy with this diet.

How will you proceed for the treatment with ketogenic diet? First of all, you have to schedule an appointment with your dietician or the medical practitioner taking care of your child.

Initially, to begin with, the regular eating habits of your child will be ascertained. Here, the dietician will assess the amount of fat, carbohydrate, protein, you child is currently taking. He will also ask you to furnish details of your child's daily activities as per his age, growth rate, and level of activity.

When your child is put on ketogenic diet, most of the energy will be derived from fat and he will also be given small amount of both protein and carbohydrate. He will be prescribed 4 meals per day. Also, as compared to adults, children will be regulated strictly and will be under tight control when it comes to eating the right kind of food.

Ketogenic diet for treating epilepsy is ideally a 4:1 ratio. It means 4 gms of fat for every 1 gm of carbohydrate and protein, which is combined together. So, if your child is prescribed a 5:1 diet plan, it means that you have to give your child 5gms of fat for every 1 gm of protein and carbohydrate combined.

However, this is not a benchmark and the ratio might differ depending on the individual requirements of the children, and the type of treatment they ought to be prescribed aside from recording the severity of the individual epilepsy cases.

As far as the effectiveness of the diet is concerned, it may take several months for the results to become evident. However, there are several instances, when parents did not have to wait for so long and the result of the diet took effect promptly.

Implementing the ketogenic diet for epilepsy

Ideally, you have to admit your child into a hospital when the diet will be implemented. This is because your child will require close monitoring. If you are starting the diet tomorrow in the hospital, you have to fast at night today starting from evening at around 6pm or 7pm. This allows enough time for the level of ketones to build up in the body. Initially, the meals will be provided in smaller amount and gradually increase as the number of days in the hospital increases. Roughly speaking, you might have to keep your child in the hospital for a period of 5 days/less or more depending on individual patient condition and requirement. Also, if there are any prescribed medicines that your child is taking, the dietician will make sure that these medicines are devoid of sugar or any ingredient that might harm the ongoing diet meal plan.

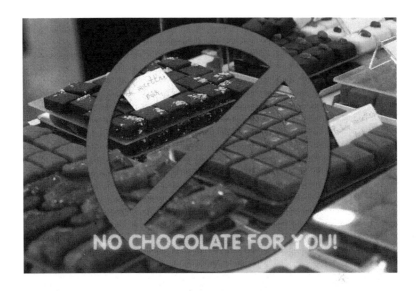

Foods that you should avoid

There are certain categories of food that you ought to stay away from. These essentially include the following-

✓ Lollies

✓ Biscuits

✓ Chocolate coated creams and cookies

✓ Sweet breads

✓ Sweetened buns

✓ Glace fruit

✓ Cakes

- ✓ Sugarless chewing gums, in addition to regular chewing gums
- ✓ Condensed milk
- ✓ Soft drinks
- ✓ Fruit juice
- ✓ Diet chocolate
- ✓ Chocolate
- ✓ Diabetic jam
- ✓ Jam
- ✓ Ice blocks
- ✓ Ice cream
- ✓ Pickles
- ✓ Sauces
- ✓ Puddings
- ✓ *Chutneys*
- ✓ Quik
- ✓ Milo
- ✓ Ovaltine
- ✓ Milk flavorings
- ✓ Pastries

✓ Pies

✓ Yogurt (flavored)

✓ Syrups and toppings

There are few important aspects that you need to be keep in mind. These are as follows-

✓ When you start the diet, you have to make sure that your child is not given any other food that deviates from the meals prescribed.

✓ The entire meal and the foods prescribed should be eaten religiously. Don't allow your child to skip meals. And it should not be the case that if your child misses protein in one meal, you will give him extra and compensate in the next meal. This is because every meal portion is calculated and worked out accordingly.

✓ No snacking is allowed in between meals. And if at all your child cannot stay without having something in between meals, you ought to talk to your dietician.

✓ If your children are of the school going age, extra care has to be taken regarding the diet outside the house. You will have to plan out the meals and the intervals or the frequency at which your child can be given the food. Seek help from the school authorities if needed. For children requiring special medical care, prescribed times of meal intake will surely be allowed by the school authorities.

✓ Don't do anything that will lower the ketone level in the body. For instance, keep him away from sugary foods. However, you can allow your child to have something made of sugar only if your child is experiencing a state called hypoglycemia, wherein the sugar levels fall very low or you can allow your child some sugar food when the level of ketones is high thereby causing discomfort and severe nausea.

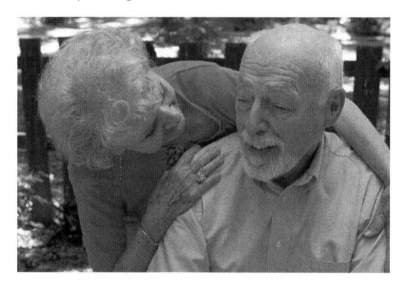

Keto diet for Alzheimer's patients

Alzheimer's disease is a neurodegenerative disorder and is oftentimes regarded as second to cancer. It is a scary disorder, which is characterized by irregular behavior patterns, failing memory, and gradual loss of the ability of organs to function in an optimum manner. This usually happens over a period of time. As the disease progresses the individual affected loses the ability to lead a normal life (walk, talk, and eat).

Although, Alzheimer's disease is a disorder that is restricted to the elderly population, individuals 60 years and above, there are several instances, when young adults between the age group of 40 and 50 are also affected. This is said to be an onset of the disease and is regarded as early stages of the deadly disease.

At the Brown University, there is a group actively involved in researching on Alzheimer's disease. They call this disease "Type 3 Diabetes". This is because there are few structural changes in the brain of the patient suffering from this ailment. Also, another factor that has contributed to calling this Type 3 Diabetes is due to the fact that the changes in the protein structure were due to development of insulin resistance over a period of time.

It has been observed that in order to work in an optimum manner, the brain cells will require glucose as source of energy. A diet that has high content of carbohydrate gives rise to increased levels of insulin and blood glucose. It is a well known fact that glucose is pushed into the neurons and this is taken care of by insulin. Over the years, owing to the fact that insulin pushes glucose into neurons, the body is not able to accept the message. As such, there is development of insulin resistance in the body.

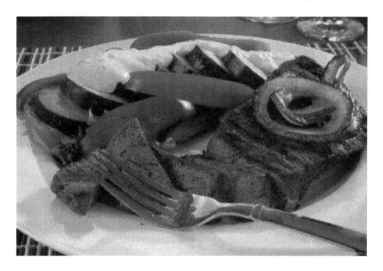

It has been observed that ketogenic diet has been able to tame this deadly disease to a great extent. Let us see how. There are several ways in which keto diet has been found to be effective in treating Alzheimer's.

✓ When you start a ketogenic diet, the number of ketones increases in the blood. So, if the brain cells have developed insulin resistance and are not being able to metabolize glucose, it can ideally make use of the ketone bodies.

✓ Insulin resistance that results over a period of time can be controlled to a great extent by adopting ketogenic diet. This not only helps brain cells from further damage but also reduces inflammation. A study that was conducted way back in the year 2012 indicates that if you are in a state of ketosis, it helps in repairing mild cognitive impairments and improves memory. Mild cognitive impairment over a period of time leads to dementia. So, you can arrest the further deterioration that leads to mild cognitive impairment too.

✓ These days coconut oil is being used for treating the disease. This is because it comprises medium chain fatty acids. These fatty acids have the ability to be stored inside the body and they can be promptly burnt for energy when needed are consumed. As a result of this action, there is production of ketones in the body, which can serve as fuel for the brain cells that are not being able to metabolize glucose due to insulin resistance. To get the best results, while treatment with coconut oil, you can use 5 tablespoons, which is equivalent to approximately 74ml of coconut oil per day. This amount can be taken per meal. And if you want to prevent Alzheimer's disease, it is recommended you take 2 to 3 tablespoons of coconut oil, which is approximately 30 ml to 44ml per day.

Role of Keto therapy in cancer treatment

More and more people are trying to adopt ketogenic diet as one of the measures to arrest progression of cancer. But as per experts it won't be long when bringing about changes in the diet could actually tame cancer cells brilliantly. When you are on a ketogenic diet, you have to take limited amount of carbohydrate, considerable amount of fat, and almost the same amount of protein.

What experts say is that cancer cells will require glucose to survive. And as we know that carbohydrates are responsible for converting glucose in your body. So, if you opt for a ketogenic diet, you are starving yourself of the carbohydrate that is generally needed on a daily basis. This will in turn impact the ability of the cancer cells to thrive and also they won't get the required energy to progress cell proliferation, which is technically known as the mTOR pathway. Also, low amount of protein has been found to be responsible in restricting the mTOR pathway to a great extent.

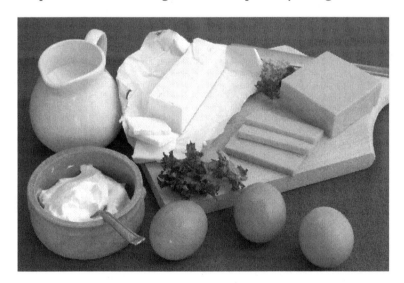

Cutting off energy to tame cancer cells

As per experts, regardless of whether you are suffering from cancer or not, it is best to switch over to ketogenic diet for almost everyone. In this way, you will be able to restrict harmful carbs and substitute them with high fat and low carb and protein. This diet will also help all those that are suffering from any kind of degenerative disease. One of the main advantages of adopting this line of treatment is that it is non toxic and the body can also adapt to burning ketone bodies for obtaining the necessary energy required for all activities.

Inhibiting cell proliferation and cell metastases

After extensive research and thoroughly studying the scenario, Professor Thomas Seyfried (Biologist) prefers to believe that unlike the common belief, cancer is not a genetic disease but it essentially is a metabolic disease. Few scientists also believe (Chris Woollams) that by opting for the ketogenic diet, cancer metastases can be stopped, progression of cancer proliferation can be arrested, and there are times when the cancer cells can be killed. There are few theories that support what the researchers and eminent scientists have claimed. There are different schools of thought and theories that support the claim that keto diet can tame cancer. So, let us find out these theories that have been mentioned below-

✓ According to one such school of thought is that cancer cells will need glucose for carrying on their activities that is cell proliferation. Also, cancer cells are not as flexible as the normal cells. So, if these cells are deprived of their nutrients that will help them in thriving, eventually these cancer cells can be killed over time. Also, since cancer cells are not flexible they won't be able to operate in the absence of glucose.

✓ It has been observed that individuals that have high levels of plasma glucose are susceptible to cancer. As such their survival chances are lowered remarkably. And the same holds true in individuals that already have cancer and have high plasma glucose levels.

✓ Another study was conducted and it was found that in case of colorectal cancer, depriving the cells of glucose produced positive results.

✓ Studies have also revealed that if you are able to reduce the intake of calories by as much as 15% on a day to day basis, the chances of surviving cancer are enhanced greatly. So, calorie restriction can yield positive results.

✓ Fasting can also help in improving your immune system but if you turn to ketogenic diet, you don't have to fast as you are already limiting your carbohydrate intake and taking in good fats, and equal amount of protein.

✓ While ketogenic diet can restrict progression of cancer cells, the moment you defy the prescribed diet, levels of glutamine, insulin, glucose, and IGF-1 gets raised.

Increased levels of glucose, glutamine, IGF-1, and insulin can again trigger the cancer cells to become active again. But when you attain ketosis, you must try to remain in ketosis. While the normal cells have the ability to derive energy by burning ketones in the event they are deprived of carbohydrates, the cancer cells cannot switch over the function and instead remain starved if they don't receive adequate carbohydrate.

The best way to stay fit and not allow cancer cells to tame you is by following these easy and simple steps. Check them out-

✓ Opt for non starchy vegetables and no other carbohydrate

✓ Keep soft drinks and glucose and fructose corn syrups at bay.

✓ Take protein in limited quantity

✓ Good fats are good for health. Bank on walnut, flaxseed, oils, olive oil, fish, avocados, coconut oil, seeds, nuts, and macadamia. Avoid trans fat.

Chapter 5

ASSESSING THE KETO DIET

What do GPs say?

An assistant professor in surgery, the ketogenic diet was first designed by Dr Gianfranco Cappello at the University of Italy. As per his study and reports, as many as 19,000 dieters derived positive results from this diet. And the best part is that these dieters experienced very few side effects and were able to remain the same without regaining weight for a considerable period of time. The ones undergoing the diet lost near about 10.2kg of weight, which is equivalent to approximately 22 pounds.

There are many GPs or medical practitioners that approve of the keto diet. For instance, Dr Oliver Di Pietro, a doctor based in Florida is encouraging individuals to opt for this diet, only at the cost of USD$1,500. According to this doctor, the ketogenic diet is safe and can benefit the ones that are looking forward to lose a few pounds and stay healthy.

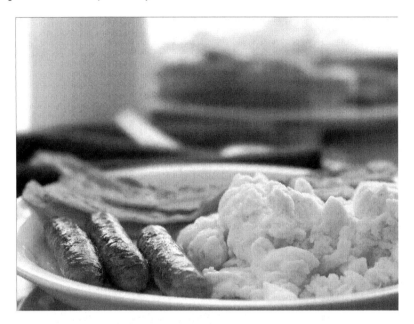

However, this form of diet has not received approval from all quarters. Different people have differing views about this form of diet. Some of the views, either for the diet or against it are mentioned below. So, read on.

✓ As per few nutritionists, the weight loss program should not be opted for as rapid weight loss causes harmful effects in the long run. Another aspect that the nutritionists objected to was that tube feeding is usually regarded as a last resort. And this form of feeding should be applicable only in the case when the patient is having mobility problem and or is on ventilator. But this kind of feeding is usually a resort that we tend to turn to at the end, when all other avenues have failed to give the desired results.

✓ Another prominent nutritionist also went on to say that keto diet comprises low carb diet and the amount of carb you are allowed to take is not more than 800 calories. So, you are literally starving yourself.

✓ Another general practitioner known as Blinten is of the opinion that a keto diet may cause injury than good to people especially if they are suffering from other ailments like kidney and liver diseases.

✓ According to Melinda Hemmelgarn, a dietician in Columbia, Missouri, says that "It's crazy to consider sticking a tube down your nose to lose weight. It sounds to me like somebody is making a lot of money on someone else's vulnerabilities. Just say no to this idea".

It goes without saying that whenever a new nutrition protocol is introduced, there is bound to be difference of opinion and while few will support the idea, few will not. The ones opposing this diet protocol does not necessarily mean that you will oppose too. Generally speaking, whenever we explain a diet or a treatment or any weight loss regime, we always mention that the results will differ depending on a number of factors that include age, weight, profession, gender, and current state of health, medication, and severity of the disease suffering from. Aside from that you will most importantly, have to take into account the rate of metabolism in each and every individual, which is bound to be different.

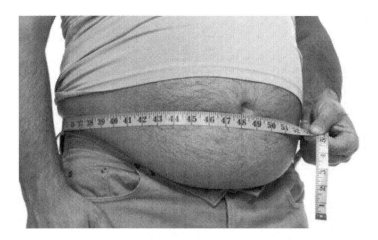

Keto diet for folks with high BMI

Whenever a new diet hits the weight watchers' group, a number of questions crop up in their minds. While few want to know whether or not the ketogenic diet will be able to help individuals stay off the diet on a long term basis, there are few that are concerned about the safety of the diet, especially if they have few other ailments like kidney and liver disorder. Similarly, there are many obese people that are worried that with their kind of BMI or Body Mass Index, whether or not the ketogenic diet will work.

Here we will discuss about just that. Body Mass Index or BMI takes into account the height and weight of the individual for calculation. If you have a BMI of 25 and more, you are regarded as "overweight". And if your BMI goes above 30, you are "obese". However this is not a reliable way of measuring the weight or the BMI as the amount of fat that is present in the body cannot be calculated. This is because on many instances, it has been observed that an athlete that is very active has a BMI that is similar to the BMI of an individual that has led a sedentary life for most of the time. As such, the results, we know are not correct. If it is found that your obesity is due to the presence of excessive fat in your body, it does not make you susceptible to ailments or you cannot be regarded as unhealthy.

Depending on your body physique, it is best to consult a medical practitioner and find out how you will need to adjust your meal plans. If the GP thinks that switching to ketogenic diet can yield better results for you, you can go ahead and opt for the same. But your BMI should not be a deciding factor alone as to whether or not you will need a special diet plan.

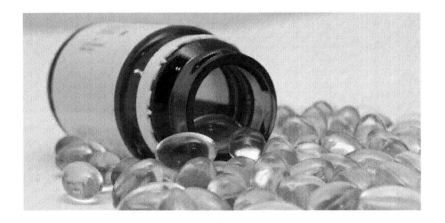

Vitamin & mineral supply

The ketogenic diet as we know comprises low carbohydrate, high fat, and sufficient amount of protein. Low amount of carbohydrate has been found to be beneficial for the ones that are looking forward to lose weight. And we know that carbohydrate is the main source of glucose. Most of the cells in the body require glucose to carry out its activities. However, this is not the case with all the cells. For instance, muscle cells can make use of protein and fat. While brain cells cannot do without glucose.

Once there is inadequate glucose in the body, which is required for all activities, the body automatically resorts to ketone bodies to get the desired energy. And in ketogenic diet, you attain a state of ketosis, wherein the number of ketone bodies in the blood is high. So, as per the diet plan, you can take only protein, high fat, and carbohydrate in a limited quantity. But vitamins and minerals are equally important for your body, especially if you are feeling weak and fatigued.

When you are on ketogenic diet, you cannot incorporate vitamins and minerals in the usual quantity that you used to prior to starting the ketogenic diet. But you can always incorporate these in limited amount. Seek assistance from your GP. He will be the best to guide you about how much vitamins and minerals you will actually need, while you are on ketogenic diet. Remember, the requirement will differ from person to person as the rate of metabolism in no 2 individuals is the same. Unless you take vitamins and minerals in your diet, you might feel fatigued and weak. You might also experience muscle weakness, which is definitely not a desirable state.

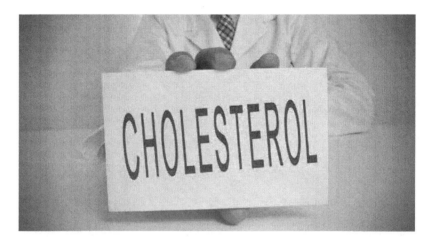

Effect of Keto on cholesterol

It goes without saying that adopting ketogenic diet means that a state called ketosis will be the outcome. Ketosis occurs because we incorporate low carbohydrate meal and adequate amount of protein along with high fat. These cause the metabolism of your body to get altered and also the manner in which energy is used up in the body changes remarkably. Experts are of the opinion that those diets that cause ketosis to result will invariably cause the level of cholesterol to go down.

Initially, when carbohydrate is allowed, only a limited amount will be permitted. This amount will be as low as 20gm per day. However, as the diet plan regime progresses, the amount of carbohydrate that was initially allowed gradually increase. Ketones are a result of ketosis. Ketone bodies are produced when fatty acids are broken down by the liver, which are used as fuel for getting the required energy. The higher the number of ketone bodies present in the blood, earlier will the state of ketosis result. As the body fat is burnt down, it impacts cholesterol in the body, which will eventually be lowered.

It may be mentioned here that levels of cholesterol in the body will be affected by the weight. Aside from this the amount of body fat you have also influences the level of cholesterol in the body.

Usually, it is seen that individuals with high cholesterol levels are also overweight or obese. Since ketogenic diet aims at helping you to lose weight over a period of time by inducing a state of ketosis, it can be safely said that if the body weight is reduced, the level of cholesterol will also go down.

Chapter 6

Is Keto Right for You?

Over the past few years, Ketogenic diet has gained a lot of momentum. Health nuts and regular folks alike are going gaga over this low carb diet. As you may have already figured out, the primary focus of Ketogenic diet is to induce the state of ketosis through lowering carbohydrate intake. Ketosis is our body's way of surviving when it receives lesser food. During ketosis, the body produces ketones, which are produced through the breakdown of fat in the liver. Through a properly designed and maintained ketogenic diet plan, you can force your body into this special metabolic state. The best thing about this diet is that it burns fat to produce energy, and you don't even have to starve to get this process started. Since our bodies are adaptive to changes, it learns to use fat storage as the primary source of energy as you lessen your carbohydrate intake and increase fat consumption.

The numerous benefits of Ketogenic diet has made it even more appealing to the crowds. The diet keeps your cholesterol in check, helps you lose weight, maintains a healthy blood sugar level, puts an end to the constant hunger pangs, and provides your body with sufficient energy. Recent studies have also shown that those who have tried this diet have experienced a significant drop in skin inflammation and acne lesions. Once you begin your keto journey, you will start to notice changes in your body. Don't be scared if you experience headaches, flu-like symptoms, mental fogginess, aggravation, dizziness and so on. Understand that your body is used to derive energy from carbohydrate. Over the period of time, the body builds a host of enzymes that helps break down carbohydrate, whereas there are only a few enzymes that deal with fat. So, when you increase fat consumption and lower glucose levels, the body has to produce enzymes to support the metabolic needs.

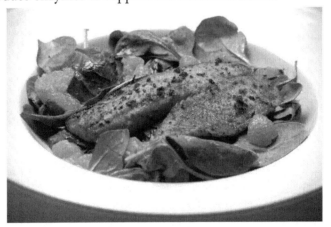

Once your body gets used to the ketogenic state, it will naturally use whatever glucose is left in your body. This means that the glycogen levels will be depleted, and this may cause a lack of energy, causing you to feel lethargic. For the first few weeks, your body will adjust to these changes, and adapt itself accordingly. Also, since ketosis tends to cause a diuretic effect, your body may be flushed out of electrolytes. T0 battle this, you need to keep yourself hydrated. Don't forget to drink plenty of water, and increase your sodium intake. So a bit of salt in your food won't necessarily hurt. In fact, it will replenish electrolytes and retain water.

However, when making the life changing decision of whether or not to adapt to the keto lifestyle, you need to ask yourself an important question – "Is keto right for me?" The ketogenic diet can be beneficial for varying groups of people. But knowing how this diet can be advantageous specifically for you and/or your family will help you be surer of your decision.

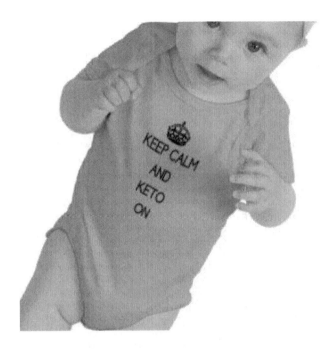

Keto diet for kids

As a parent, you always want what's best for your kids, especially when it comes to nutrition. So, when choosing a diet plan that is not conventional, you may wonder if that is the right choice for you to make. Research shows that ketogenic diet has been especially beneficial for children suffering from epileptic seizures and childhood obesity. Since the 1920's, ketogenic diet has been used as an alternative therapy for epilepsy in children. When the antiepileptic drugs used to fail to control the intractable seizures, doctors would resort to dietary therapies. In a retrospective study, growth and biochemical data were collected from around 12 children, who belonged to the ages of 3-4 years and were on ketogenic diet for 6 months. 90% of their caloric intake came from fat, whereas only 10% came from carbohydrate/protein along with additional minerals and vitamins. After a thorough analysis of the biochemical data, it was found that all children demonstrated fewer numbers of seizures. The diet had caused no significant side effect or interruption in normal growth of the children over the 6 month time period. Thus, the diet seemed to be safe both in terms of laboratory parameters and growth.

Ketogenic diet has also been proven to be helpful for children of any age with atonic (drop), absence, and myoclonic seizures. Babies can also receive this diet through a specially made formula. Doctors often prescribe this diet for babies with grand-mal (tonic-clonic) seizures. When medicines don't work or cause unnecessary side-effects, ketogenic diet can be used as an alternative therapy.

Also, when it comes to childhood obesity, the best way to beat it is to cut down on the sugar and starch intake. New studies show that children (of the age of 13 and above) can lose significant weight simply by following a low-carb diet. On the other hand, children who were on a low-fat, low-calorie diet struggled to lose weight despite feeling hungry all the time. Aside from helping kids lose weight, ketogenic diet also improves their overall health. If you want a smart diet that will keep your little one fit and healthy, a low-carb and high fat diet is the way to go!

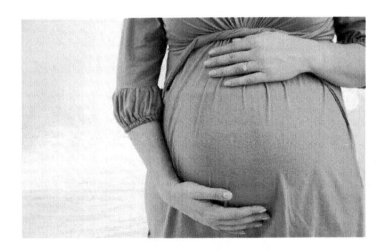

Keto nutrition during pregnancy

So you are thinking of adapting to the keto lifestyle, but you are not sure if you should continue during pregnancy. Well, you are not alone in this dire predicament. With the ever increasing popularity of ketogenic diet, women all over the world are getting more inclined to swear by the high fat, low-carb diet. However, questions are being raised about how safe this diet is for would be mothers. If you are new to this lifestyle, you might start to second guess your decision as soon as you get to know about the opposing views people have about ketogenic diet. However, you should know that a low carb diet is proven to be helpful for women dealing with infertility. Since there is a lot of debate going on about whether or not ketogenic diet is a healthy dietary alternative for pregnant women, you may find a lot of doctors advising against it. However, when you mention that your diet will consist of eggs, meat, fish, fresh vegetables, dairy, seeds, nuts and a little bit of fruits, they may readily agree to it because of the nutritional value of all the things you will be consuming.

The controversy over ketogenic diet arises from the misconceptions that people have about ketosis and how it affects the body. Despite being incorrect, the misconception that ketosis is harmful for the fetus is widely popular. However, research shows that ketosis is actually favorable to pregnant women. When compared to non-pregnant women, it was found that blood ketone concentration is about 3 times higher in pregnant women after overnight fasts. Also, during the later stages of pregnancy, metabolism turns into a state of catabolism when ketosis is even more frequent. In light of this information, it would be safe to say that pregnant women, regardless of what type of diet they are on, would experience ketosis at some stage of their pregnancy (especially if she experiences food aversion or nausea).

The misconception that ketosis is harmful for the developing baby seems illogical. For example, nutritional ketosis leads to normal blood sugar levels, normal acid balance, and low levels of blood ketones. So, if you consume a low-carb diet during pregnancy, you may experience ketosis from time to time, but it won't be anywhere close to DKA or Diabetic ketoacidosis, which is harmful and occurs in people who are insulin dependent diabetic. DKA occurs when a diabetic individual skips their insulin shots or takes the incorrect dosage. In case of a non-diabetic pregnant woman, even if she tests positive for urinary ketones, the chances are highly likely that her blood ketones levels would be very low.

Despite all that is being said about the harmful effects of ketogenic diet on the fetus, studies show that the fetal brain receives about 30% of the energy from ketones. In fact, ketones are necessary for the growing fetus when synthesizing a range of essential cerebral lipids. This is another reason behind the occurrence of ketosis during the third trimester. Also, most importantly, ketones are so vital that the fetus itself manufactures ketones on its own. Blood samples taken from the umbilical veins indicate higher levels of ketones. So as it turns out, the fetus needs ketones as much as it needs glucose for growth. Providing fuel in excess may be harmful. However, if you consume sufficient calories and maintain healthy blood sugar levels, your baby will get the right mix.

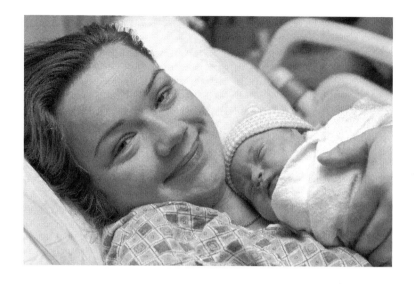

Keto for breastfeeding mothers

Pregnancy and childbirth changes your body in ways you may not have predicted. You may want to get back to shape as soon as you walk out of the hospital with your beautiful baby in your arms. However, remember that the weight you have put on during pregnancy did not occur overnight. So, you cannot expect to disappear right away either. You cannot throw yourself into strenuous workout right after childbirth. However, there is a way to lose weight and feel healthy simply by keeping your diet in check. Ketogenic diet has been designed to provide nursing mothers ample nutrition, while also allowing their bodies to get back to shape. A low carb, high protein diet can be a boon for your body post childbirth. However, you would have to do it in the right manner. If you have never tried the ketogenic diet before, you must not delve into it right after childbirth. Your body will need time to adjust its metabolism according to the changes in your diet. So, taking it slow and in a step by step manner would be wise.

Studies show that human babies experience ketosis soon after birth, and they remain in that state even during the nursing stages. Babies use fats and ketones for brain growth and energy. Remember that babies are not in ketosis right after birth. There is a brief delay before the process starts. Researchers believe that the delay in ketogenesis may occur due to limited supply of carnitine, which comes from milk. It was also found that gluconeogenesis and glycogenolysis (the process in which glucose is derived from protein) do not occur immediately. This way, it would be safe to say even though ketogenesis takes time to kick in, the process known as keto-adaption starts right after.

The reason some researchers believe that ketogenic metabolism is desirable while breastfeeding is because newborns can thrive from the nutrition they will get from the milk. In spite of the moderate sugar levels in the breast milk, breastfeeding can be considered ketogenic. The period right after birth is crucial for the baby's growth and extensive brain growth takes place during this phase. Although the composition of the breast milk may be affected by the diet, it is safe to assume that breast milk has always been ketogenic. Not only does a ketogenic diet boost the baby's brain growth, but it also fights a variety of brain disorders.

Despite everything that has been said in favor of ketogenic diet while breastfeeding, it would be safer for you maintain certain precautions to make sure everything goes smoothly. Keeping your diet in the "maintenance mode" will give your body time to adjust to the new change in diet, which will be healthy for both you and your baby. So, in the beginning stages, you can keep your carbohydrate levels close to 100 grams a day, and you can slowly reduce that amount to no more than 25 grams a day. This way, the change won't be drastic, and it would take place naturally. For all the newbies out there, here are a few more tips that you should follow when adapting to the keto diet during the nursing stage:

Wait till your newborn is 2-6 months old before beginning the diet

- ✓ Don't decrease your carbohydrate intake drastically all of a sudden
- ✓ Keep your caloric intake in check
- ✓ Drink plenty of water
- ✓ Watch out for your milk supply
- ✓ Track your baby's diaper output and watch their weight

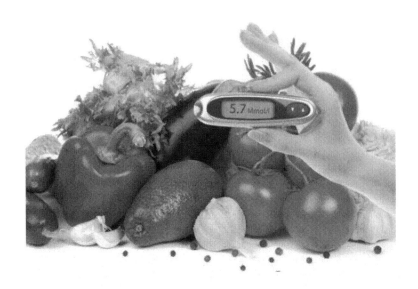

What about diabetics?

Diabetes is a difficult disease that afflicts over 26 million Americans. It is accompanied by a chain of other health scares, and also challenges the quality of the life of the sufferer. Scientists have been looking for smarter ways to beat this disease, and researchers believe that the ketogenic diet could part of the solution. This diet has been around for a long time now, and it is traced back to the 1920s. Back in those days when injectable insulin was not developed, ketogenic diet was used to curb this malicious disease. Since then the diet has been examined and evaluated to see if it really is beneficial for diabetic individuals. Today, despite opposition, a group of researchers and nutrition experts believe that the keto diet may revolutionize the way diabetes is treated.

Although the ADA (American Diabetes Association) recommends 135 grams of carbs per day, the ketogenic diet restricts daily carb intake to 20 grams. When following the keto diet, you need to consume 80% fat and only 20% carbs/proteins. As stated by the Keto diet community, the diet mimics various aspects of starvation by forcing our body to burn fats instead of carbohydrate for energy. Once ketosis occurs and the liver produces ketone bodies, glucose is replaced by these ketone bodies as the body's primary energy source. A recent study conducted by the Kuwait University shows that the keto diet significantly improves the diabetic state and stabilizes hyperglycemia. Thus, by following a keto diet, glucose levels can be brought down to a near normal state.

A study published in the Nutrition and Metabolism journal revealed that when tried on 21 people with type 2 diabetes, the ketogenic diet improved their blood sugar levels by 16% on average over a 16 weeks time period. More than 6% of the participants reached their desired weight, and over 17% of the participants were able to reduce or discontinue their diabetes meds. The ketogenic diet may seem like a carnivorous' dream, but there are restrictions to follow. If you are wishing to try out this diet, make sure you consult your doctor first about how you should proceed.

Chapter 7

MAKING YOUR JOURNEY EASIER

Changing your diet completely and going for a low carb, high fat diet is not going to be an easy transition. When you start on ketogenic diet, you would have to maintain a healthy balance of 80% fat and 20% protein/carb. Even if your favorite meals consist of cakes and ice creams, you would have to curb such desires when you adapt to the keto lifestyle. Staying determined and sticking to your diet plan may seem difficult at first. However, your journey can be made easier with the right plan and guidance. Here are few tips that you would find to be helpful:

✓ Eat less than 20 grams of net carbs every day to get into ketosis.

✓ Get yourself some ketostix. These are inexpensive, and you can even cut into half.

✓ Eat enough salt.

✓ Drink enough water. Don't go easy on your fluids. Drink as much water as you can so you don't get dehydrated.

✓ Read labels before trying out any new product. They may contain ingredients that you should avoid when on a keto diet.

✓ Include a cup of chicken broth in your meals.

✓ Skip exercising for the first weeks.

✓ Get to know as much as you can about ketosis and ketogenic diet.

If you want to carry on with your ketogenic diet plan successfully, you would need to be honest with it. Don't give into temptation, and avoid those "cheat days" when you let yourself enjoy higher amounts of carbs. You may even consult a nutritionist to help you sketch a proper diet plan for you.

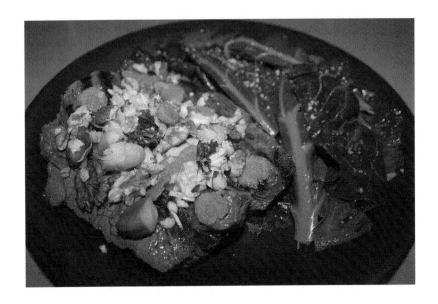

2 Weeks meal plan furnished for you

When starting something new, we all need a bit of guidance. The same applies to when you are trying out a new diet. In order to make things easier for you, here I present a 2-week meal plan that you can go through to understand how you can plan your meals. You can either make your meal plans at the beginning of every week, or before beginning a new month. The choice is yours. Here's a 14-day meal plan including breakfast, lunch and dinner. You will find the recipes of these delicious meals in the next chapter!

Day 1

Breakfast:

Zucchini Breakfast Hash

- ✓ **Total carbs:** 9.1 gm

- ✓ Fiber: 2.5 gm

- ✓ **Net carbs:** 6.6 gm

- ✓ Fat: 35.5 gm

- ✓ Protein: 17.4 gm

- ✓ Calories: 422 kcal

- ✓ Potassium:775mg

- ✓ Magnesium: 53mg

Lunch:

Easter Frittata

- ✓ **Total carbs:** 10.1 gm

- ✓ Fiber: 3.5 gm

- ✓ **Net carbs:** 6.6 gm

- ✓ Fat: 37.5 gm

✓ Protein: 25.5 gm

✓ Potassium: 625 mg

✓ Magnesium: 40 mg

✓ Calories: 504 kcal

Dinner:

Salmon with Creamy Spinach & Hollandaise Sauce

✓ **Total carbs:** 6.5 gm

✓ Fiber: 2.8 gm

✓ **Net carbs:** 3.7 gm

✓ Fat: 72.6 gm

✓ Protein: 34 gm

✓ Potassium: 1314 mg

✓ Magnesium: 143 mg

✓ Calories: 813 kcal

Day 2

Breakfast:

All Day Ketogenic Breakfast

- ✓ **Total carbs:** 15.5 gm

- ✓ Fiber: 8.9 gm

- ✓ **Net carbs:** 6.6 gm

- ✓ Fat: 41.3 gm

- ✓ Protein: 19.5 gm

- ✓ Potassium: 1307 mg

- ✓ Magnesium: 43 mg

- ✓ Calories: 489 kcal

Lunch:

Low-carb Mediterranean Risotto

- ✓ **Total carbs:** 10.2 gm

- ✓ Fiber: 4 gm

- ✓ **Net carbs:** 6.2 gm

- ✓ Fat: 33.4 gm

✓ Protein: 41 gm

✓ Potassium: 1113 mg

✓ Magnesium: 78 mg

✓ Calories: 504 kcal

Dinner:

Easter Frittata

✓ **Total carbs:** 10.1 gm

✓ Fiber: 3.5 gm

✓ **Net carbs:** 6.6 gm

✓ Fat: 37.5 gm

✓ Protein: 25.5 gm

✓ Potassium: 625 mg

✓ Magnesium: 40 mg

✓ Calories: 504 kcal

Day 3

Breakfast:

Pesto Scrambled Eggs

- ✓ **Total carbs:** 3.3 gm

- ✓ Fiber: 0.7 gm

- ✓ **Net carbs:** 2.6 gm

- ✓ Fat: 41.5 g

- ✓ Protein: 20.4 gm

- ✓ Potassium: 327 mg

- ✓ Magnesium: 25 mg

- ✓ Calories: 467 kcal

Lunch:

Keto Bun with Avocado & Bacon

- ✓ **Total carbs:** 24.1 gm

- ✓ Fiber: 16.2 gm

- ✓ **Net carbs:** 8 gm

- ✓ Fat: 61.5 gm

✓ Protein: 17.4 gm

✓ Potassium: 1155 mg

✓ Magnesium: 131 mg

✓ Calories: 673 kcal

Dinner:

Low-carb Mediterranean Risotto

✓ **Total carbs:** 10.2 gm

✓ Fiber: 4 gm

✓ **Net carbs:** 6.2 gm

✓ Fat: 33.4 g

✓ Protein: 41 g

✓ Potassium: 1113 mg

✓ Magnesium: 78 mg

✓ Calories: 504 kcal

Day 4

Breakfast:

Vanilla Keto Smoothie

- ✓ **Total carbs:** 5.6 gm

- ✓ Fiber: 0.5 gm

- ✓ **Net carbs:** 5.1 gm

- ✓ Fat: 45.2 gm

- ✓ Protein: 34.6 g

- ✓ Potassium: 598 mg

- ✓ Magnesium: 26 mg

- ✓ Calories: 566 kcal

Lunch:

Paleo Styled Stuffed Avocado

- ✓ **Total carbs:** 19.5 gm

- ✓ Fiber: 14 gm

- ✓ **Net carbs:** 5.5 gm

- ✓ Fat: 52.6 gm

✓ Protein: 27.2 gm

✓ Potassium: 1410 mg

✓ Magnesium: 99 mg

✓ Calories: 633 kcal

Dinner:

Keto Mexican Rice

✓ **Total carbs:** 10.1 gm

✓ Fiber: 3.7 gm

✓ **Net carbs:** 6.4 gm

✓ Fat: 31 gm

✓ Protein: 17.6 gm

✓ Potassium: 763 mg

✓ Magnesium: 39 mg

✓ Calories: 385 kcal

Day 5

Breakfast:

Chocolate Chia Pudding

- ✓ **Total carbs:** 21.2 gm

- ✓ Fiber: 14.9 gm

- ✓ **Net carbs:** 6.3 gm

- ✓ Fat: 26.6 gm

- ✓ Protein: 9.5 gm

- ✓ Potassium: 364 mg

- ✓ Magnesium: 63 mg

- ✓ Calories: 329 kcal

Lunch:

Keto Mexican Rice

- ✓ **Total carbs:** 10.1 gm

- ✓ Fiber: 3.7 gm

- ✓ **Net carbs:** 6.4 gm

- ✓ Fat: 31 gm

- ✓ Protein: 17.6 gm

- ✓ Potassium: 763 mg

- ✓ Magnesium: 39 mg

- ✓ Calories: 385 kcal

Dinner:

Ribeye Steak with Gremolata served with Creamy Mash

- ✓ **Total carbs:** 12.7 gm

- ✓ Fiber: 4.4 gm

- ✓ **Net carbs:** 8.3 gm

- ✓ Fat: 90.2 gm

- ✓ Protein: 41.7 gm

- ✓ Potassium: 1477 mg

- ✓ Magnesium: 97 mg

- ✓ Calories: 1024 kcal

Day 6

Breakfast:

Pesto Scrambled Eggs

✓ **Total carbs:** 3.3 gm

✓ Fiber: 0.7 gm

✓ **Net carbs:** 2.6 gm

✓ Fat: 41.5 gm

✓ Protein: 20.4 gm

✓ Potassium: 327 mg

✓ Magnesium: 25 mg

✓ Calories: 467 kcal

Lunch:

Keto Mexican Rice

✓ **Total carbs:** 10.1 gm

✓ Fiber: 3.7 gm

✓ **Net carbs:** 6.4 gm

✓ Fat: 31 g

✓ Protein: 17.6 g

✓ Potassium: 763 mg

✓ Magnesium: 39 mg

✓ Calories: 385 kcal

Dinner:

Pork Chops Served with Creamy Keto Mash

- ✓ **Total carbs:** 10.9 gm
- ✓ Fiber: 3.9 gm
- ✓ **Net carbs:** 7 gm
- ✓ Fat: 56.5 gm
- ✓ Protein: 34.4 gm
- ✓ Potassium: 1110 mg
- ✓ Magnesium: 66 mg
- ✓ Calories: 690 kcal

Day 7

Breakfast:

Pumpkin Pie Chia Pudding

- ✓ **Total carbs:** 20.8 gm
- ✓ Fiber: 14.2 gm
- ✓ **Net carbs:** 6.6 gm
- ✓ Fat: 22.4 gm

✓ Protein: 8.1 gm

✓ Potassium: 283 mg

✓ Magnesium: 39 mg

✓ Calories: 295 kcal

Lunch:

Pork Chops Served with Creamy Keto Mash

✓ **Total carbs:** 10.9 gm

✓ Fiber: 3.9 gm

✓ **Net carbs:** 7 gm

✓ Fat: 56.5 gm

✓ Protein: 34.4 gm

✓ Potassium: 1110 mg

✓ Magnesium: 66 mg

✓ Calories: 690 kcal

Dinner:

Paleo Styled Stuffed Avocado

✓ **Total carbs: 19.5 gm**

   ✓ Fiber: 14 gm

✓ **Net carbs: 5.5 gm**

   ✓ Fat: 52.6 gm

   ✓ Protein: 27.2 gm

   ✓ Potassium: 1410 mg

   ✓ Magnesium: 99 mg

   ✓ Calories: 633 kcal

Day 8

Breakfast:

Brussels Sprout with Bacon Hash

✓ **Total carbs: 11.6 gm**

   ✓ Fiber: 4.5 gm

✓ **Net carbs: 7.1 gm**

  ✓ Fat: 20 gm

  ✓ Protein: 20 gm

  ✓ Potassium: 809 mg

  ✓ Magnesium: 45 mg

  ✓ Calories: 31.6 kcal

Lunch:

Keto Bun with Avocado & Bacon

✓ **Total carbs: 24.1 gm**

  ✓ Fiber: 16.2 gm

✓ **Net carbs: 8 gm**

  ✓ Fat: 61.5 gm

  ✓ Protein: 17.4 gm

  ✓ Potassium: 1155 mg

  ✓ Magnesium: 131 mg

  ✓ Calories: 673 kcal

Dinner:

Cajun Chicken Tacos

✓ **Total carbs: 9 gm**

   ✓ Fiber: 2.6 gm

✓ **Net carbs: 6.4 gm**

   ✓ Fat: 35.4 gm

   ✓ Protein: 40.6 gm

   ✓ Potassium: 816 mg

   ✓ Magnesium: 70 mg

   ✓ Calories: 521 kcal

Day 9

Breakfast:

Keto Mexican Chocolate Shake

✓ **Total carbs: 14.4 gm**

   ✓ Fiber: 8.2 gm

✓ Net carbs: 6.2 gm

- ✓ Fat: 52.1 gm

- ✓ Protein: 6 gm

- ✓ Potassium: 385 mg

- ✓ Magnesium: 75 mg

- ✓ Calories: 503 kcal

Lunch:

Cajun Chicken Tacos

✓ Total carbs: 9 gm

- ✓ Fiber: 2.6 gm

✓ Net carbs: 6.4 gm

- ✓ Fat: 35.4 gm

- ✓ Protein: 40.6 gm

- ✓ Potassium: 816 mg

- ✓ Magnesium: 70 mg

- ✓ Calories: 521 kcal

Dinner:

Pan-roasted salmon Served with green beans

✓ **Total carbs: 11.1 gm**

   ✓ Fiber: 3.8 gm

✓ **Net carbs: 7.3 gm**

   ✓ Fat: 33.8 gm

   ✓ Protein: 36 gm

   ✓ Potassium: 956 mg

   ✓ Magnesium: 91 mg

   ✓ Calories: 489 kcal

Day 10

Breakfast:

Vanilla Keto Smoothie

✓ **Total carbs: 5.6 gm**

   ✓ Fiber: 0.5 gm

✓ ## Net carbs: 5.1 gm

- ✓ Fat: 45.2 gm

- ✓ Protein: 34.6 gm

- ✓ Potassium: 598 mg

- ✓ Magnesium: 26 mg

- ✓ Calories: 566 kcal

Lunch:

Avocado Salad served with 2 tbsp mayonnaise or vinaigrette

✓ ## Total carbs: 22.2 gm

- ✓ Fiber: 15.5 gm

✓ ## Net carbs: 6.7 gm

- ✓ Fat: 65.6 gm

- ✓ Protein: 14.2 gm

- ✓ Potassium: 1522 mg

- ✓ Magnesium: 109 mg

- ✓ Calories: 699 kcal

Dinner:

Spicy Cauliflower Soup Served with Keto Bun

✓ ## Total carbs: 22.9 gm

   ✓ Fiber: 11.7 gm

✓ ## Net carbs: 11.2 gm

   ✓ Fat: 34.3 gm

   ✓ Protein: 20.8 gm

   ✓ Potassium: 1080 mg

   ✓ Magnesium: 129 mg

   ✓ Calories: 459 kcal

Day 11

Breakfast:

All Day Keto Breakfast

✓ ## Total carbs: 15.5 gm

   ✓ Fiber: 8.9 gm

✓ # Net carbs: 6.6 gm

- ✓ Fat: 41.3 gm
- ✓ Protein: 19.5 gm
- ✓ Potassium: 1307 mg
- ✓ Magnesium: 43 mg
- ✓ Calories: 489 kcal

Lunch:

Spicy Cauliflower Soup Served with Keto Bun

✓ # Total carbs: 22.9 gm

- ✓ Fiber: 11.7 gm

✓ # Net carbs: 11.2 gm

- ✓ Fat: 34.3 gm
- ✓ Protein: 20.8 gm
- ✓ Potassium: 1080 mg
- ✓ Magnesium: 129 mg
- ✓ Calories: 459 kcal

Dinner:

Salmon Served with Creamy Spinach and Hollandaise Sauce

✓ **Total carbs: 6.5 gm**

   ✓ Fiber: 2.8 gm

✓ **Net carbs: 3.7 gm**

   ✓ Fat: 72.6 gm

   ✓ Protein: 34 gm

   ✓ Potassium: 1314 mg

   ✓ Magnesium: 143 mg

   ✓ Calories: 813 kcal

Day 12

Breakfast:

Pesto Scrambled Eggs

✓ **Total carbs: 3.3 gm**

   ✓ Fiber: 0.7 gm

✓ ## Net carbs: 2.6 gm

- ✓ Fat: 41.5 gm

- ✓ Protein: 20.4 gm

- ✓ Potassium: 327 mg

- ✓ Magnesium: 25 mg

- ✓ Calories: 467 kcal

Lunch:

Spicy Cauliflower Soup Served with Keto Bun

✓ ## Total carbs: 22.9 gm

- ✓ Fiber: 11.7 gm

✓ ## Net carbs: 11.2 gm

- ✓ Fat: 34.3 gm

- ✓ Protein: 20.8 gm

- ✓ Potassium: 1080 mg

- ✓ Magnesium: 129 mg

- ✓ Calories: 459 kcal

Dinner:

Spicy Chorizo Meatballs Served with Buttered Brussels Sprouts and Keto Cheese Sauce or Keto Cheese Sauce

✓ Total carbs: 17.6 gm

- ✓ Fiber: 6.6 gm

✓ Net carbs: 11 gm

- ✓ Fat: 49.5 gm

- ✓ Protein: 31.8 gm

- ✓ Potassium: 1029 mg

- ✓ Magnesium: 92 mg

- ✓ Calories: 627 kcal

Day 13

Breakfast:

Berry Chia Pudding

✓ **Total carbs: 20.3 gm**

   ✓ Fiber: 14.5 gm

✓ **Net carbs: 5.8 gm**

   ✓ Fat: 22.4 gm

   ✓ Protein: 7.9 gm

   ✓ Potassium: 230 mg

   ✓ Magnesium: 36 mg

   ✓ Calories: 288 kcal

Lunch:

Spicy Chorizo Meatballs Served with Keto Cheese Sauce or Buttered Brussels Sprouts

✓ **Total carbs: 17.6 gm**

   ✓ Fiber: 6.6 gm

✓ **Net carbs: 11 gm**

   ✓ Fat: 49.5 gm

   ✓ Protein: 31.8 gm

✓ Potassium: 1029 mg

✓ Magnesium: 92 mg

✓ Calories: 627 kcal

Dinner:

Beef Ragù with "Zoodles"

✓ **Total carbs: 8.3 gm**

✓ Fiber: 2.6 gm

✓ **Net carbs: 5.7 gm**

✓ Fat: 51.1 gm

✓ Protein: 37.8 gm

✓ Potassium: 1191 mg

✓ Magnesium: 83 mg

✓ Calories: 645 kcal

Day 14

Breakfast:

Keto Mexican Chocolate Shake

✓ ## Total carbs: 14.4 gm

   ✓ Fiber: 8.2 gm

✓ ## Net carbs: 6.2 gm

   ✓ Fat: 52.1 gm

   ✓ Protein: 6 gm

   ✓ Potassium: 385 mg

   ✓ Magnesium: 75 mg

   ✓ Calories: 503 kcal

Lunch:

Beef Ragù with "Zoodles"

✓ ## Total carbs: 8.3 gm

   ✓ Fiber: 2.6 gm

✓ **Net carbs: 5.7 gm**

- ✓ Fat: 51.1 gm

- ✓ Protein: 37.8 gm

- ✓ Potassium: 1191 mg

- ✓ Magnesium: 83 mg

- ✓ Calories: 645 kcal

Dinner:

Pan-roasted salmon and green beans

✓ **Total carbs: 11.1 gm**

- ✓ Fiber: 3.8 gm

✓ **Net carbs: 7.3 gm**

- ✓ Fat: 33.8 gm

- ✓ Protein: 36 gm

- ✓ Potassium: 956 mg

- ✓ Magnesium: 91 mg

- ✓ Calories: 489 kcal

Easy recipes that make you say yum!

In today's busy world, no one can afford to spend hours in the kitchen. When juggling professional and personal responsibilities, one wishes for quick and easy recipes that will not only be time saving, but will also be appetizing for the whole family. Whether you are cooking for just one or the family, these delectable keto recipes will surely make your life easier.

Breakfast Recipes

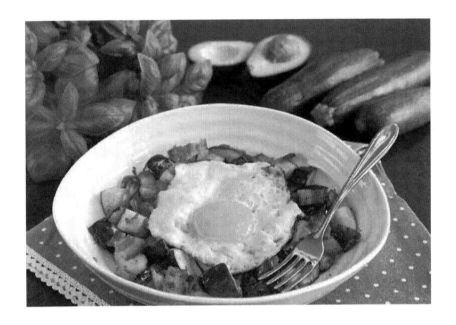

1. Zucchini Breakfast Hash

Ingredients (for 1 serving):

- ✓ 1 medium 200gm zucchini
- ✓ 2 slices of bacon about 60gms
- ✓ ½ of a small white onion about 30gms or 1 clove garlic
- ✓ 1 tbsp coconut oil or ghee

✓ 1 tbsp freshly chopped chives or parsley

✓ ¼ tsp salt

✓ 1 large egg (organic or free-range)

Instructions:

1. Start with peeling the onion or garlic and then finely chop it. After that, slice the bacon.

2. Sweat the garlic or onion over medium heat, and add the chopped bacons. Keep stirring until the ingredients have taken a light brown shade.

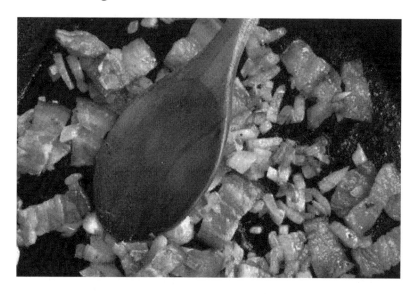

3. While the bacons and onions are frying, you can slice the zucchini into medium pieces.

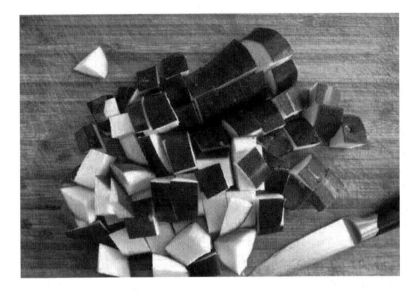

4. Add the zucchini to the frying pan and cook for about 10 to 15 minutes. When cooked, turn off the heat and add the chopped parsley or chives.

5. Serve with a fried egg on top. In case you are not allowed to have eggs, top with avocado!

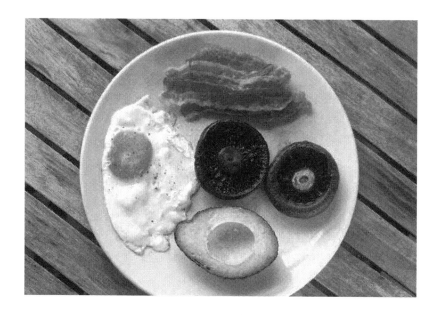

2. All Day Ketogenic Breakfast

Ingredients (for 1 serving):

- ✓ 1 large egg (organic or free-range)

- ✓ 2-3 regular or 5 think bacon rashers about 60gms

- ✓ 2 large Portobello mushrooms about 170gms

- ✓ ½ of an average avocado about 100gms

- ✓ 1 tbsp ghee or butter

- ✓ Pinch of freshly ground black pepper

✓ Salt

✓ Fresh herbs for garnishing

Instructions:

1. Start by pan roasting the mushrooms with top-side down. Heat a non sticky pan and add half of the butter or ghee over medium low heat. Add the mushrooms and then sprinkle some salt and pepper over it. Cook for about 5-9 minutes until the mushrooms are tender. Since mushroom may release some water, it would be better to fry the egg on a different pan with ghee or butter.

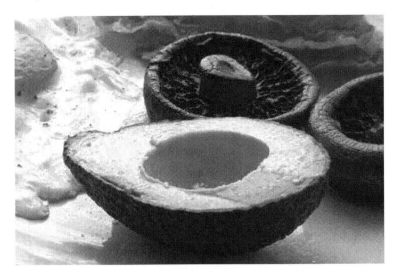

2. Although the basic meal is ready, you should add the avocado to it simply because it is healthy and it will keep you full

for few good hours. Having half of an average sized avocado should be enough. Get ready to enjoy!

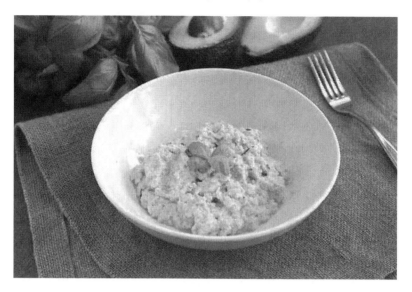

3. Pesto Scrambled Eggs

Ingredients (for 1 serving):

✓ 3 large eggs (organic or free-range)

✓ 1 tbsp of butter or ghee

✓ 1 tbsp of pesto about 15gms

✓ 2 tbsp of soured cream or crème fraîche about 30gms

✓ Salt and freshly ground black pepper

Instructions:

1. Start by cracking the eggs in a mixing bowl followed by a pinch of salt and black pepper. Beat them well with a fork or whisk.

2. Pour the beaten eggs into a pan, add the ghee or butter and turn on the heat.

3. Keep stirring the eggs over low heat so that it doesn't get dry. Then add the pesto and mix it well.

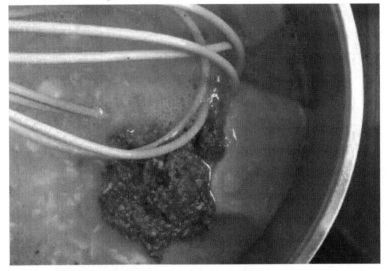

4. Turn off the heat, and add a spoonful of crème fraîche/soured cream and mix well. This will allow the egg to cool down, while maintaining its creamy texture.

5. Serve with sliced avocado on the top!

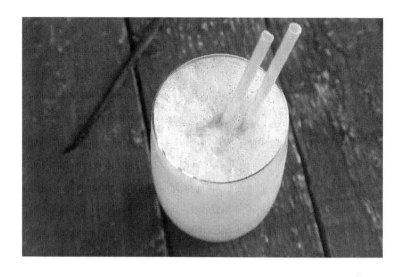

4. Vanilla Keto Smoothie

Ingredients (for 1 serving):

✓   2 large eggs or 2 tbsp of coconut butter or 2 tbsp of chia seeds

✓   ½ cup coconut milk or soured cream about 115gms

✓   ¼ cup egg white protein powder or whey protein about 25gms

✓   1 tbsp of extra virgin coconut oil or MCT oil

✓   1 tsp of vanilla extract or 1 vanilla bean

✓   3-5 drops of Stevia extract

✓   ½ cup ice + ¼ cup water

Instructions:

1. Start by adding the eggs, soured cream, egg protein powder, vanilla, stevia, water and ice into the blender. Pulse until it is smooth, and serve immediately!

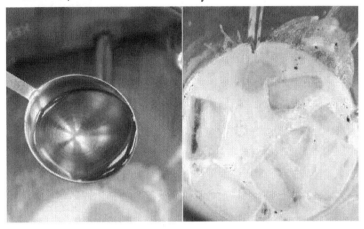

You can either use sugar-free vanilla extract, or you can go for vanilla beans. You can use either egg white protein powder or whey protein. All of these leave a great taste. If you don't like the taste of raw eggs, you can go for coconut butter or chia seeds instead.

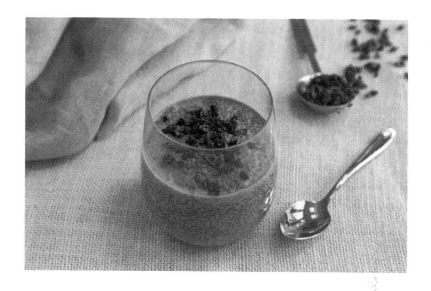

5. Chocolate Chia Pudding

Ingredients (for 1 serving):

✓ ¼ cup of chia seeds about 32gms

✓ ¼ cup of coconut milk about 60 ml

✓ ½ cup of almond milk or water about 120 ml

✓ 1 tbsp of raw unsweetened cacao powder

✓ 1 tbsp of Swerve or Erythritol about 10gms

✓ 5-10 drops of Stevia extract

✓ ½ tbsp extra dark chocolate for topping

✓ ¼ tsp of cayenne pepper and ¼ of tsp cinnamon (optional)

Instructions:

1. Start by mixing the coconut milk, chia seeds, cacao powder, water, stevia and Erythritol. If you like a smoother texture, you can place the mixture into a grinder and pulse until it becomes smooth. Sit the mixture in the fridge for 15 minutes at least, although ideally it should be overnight.

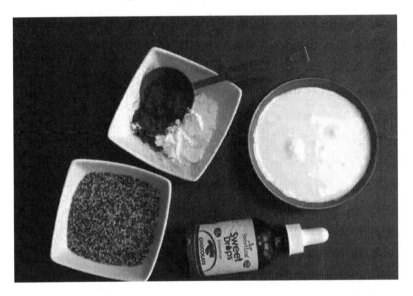

2. Take the pudding out of the fridge and top it with extra dark chocolate or cocoa nibs just before serving. Enjoy!

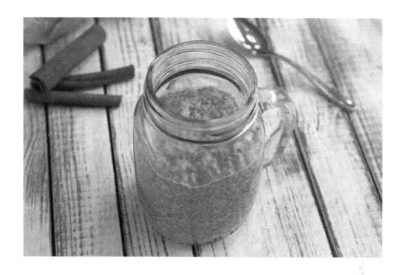

6. Pumpkin Pie Chia Pudding

Ingredients (for 1 serving):

✓   ¼ cup of chia seeds about 32gms

✓   ¼ cup of coconut milk or heavy whipped cream about 60ml

✓   ¼ cup of almond milk or water about 60 ml

✓   ¼ cup of pumpkin purée about 50gms

✓   1 tbsp of Swerve or Erythritol about 10gms

✓   5-10 drops of Stevia extract

✓   ½ tsp of gingerbread or pumpkin pie spice mix

Instructions:

1. Start by mixing chia seeds, water, coconut milk, and pumpkin pie, ½ tsp of pumpkin pie spice, stevia and Erythritol. If you like a smoother texture, make sure you use ground chia seeds.

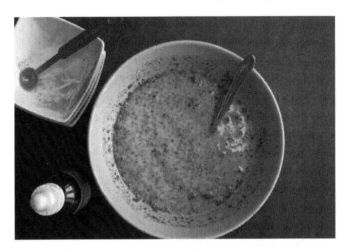

2. Transfer the mixture into a jar, and let that sit for 15 minutes in the fridge. You can also refrigerate it overnight for better taste. Take the pudding out of the fridge and top it off with pumpkin spice just before serving!

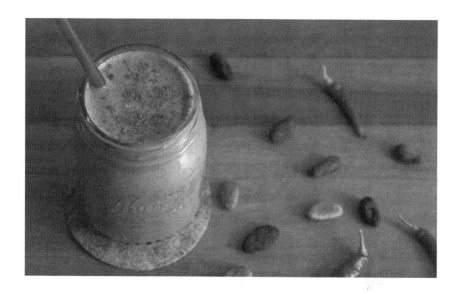

7. Keto Mexican Chocolate Shake

Ingredients (for 1 serving):

✓ ¼ cup of coconut cream about 80 ml

✓ 2 tbsp of extra virgin coconut oil

✓ 1 tbsp of ground chia seeds

✓ 2 tbsp of unsweetened cocoa powder about 10gms

✓ ¼ tsp of organic vanilla extract

✓ ¼ tsp of cinnamon powder

✓ ¼ tsp of cayenne powder

✓ 1 cup water

✓ Ice as desired

Instructions:

Mix all the ingredients and pulse it in a blender for about 1 minute. Get ready to serve and enjoy! Does it get any easier?

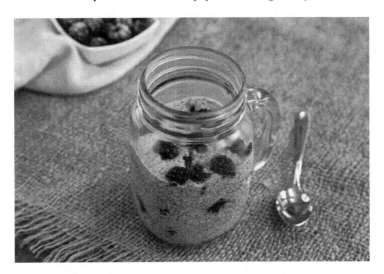

8. Berry Chia Pudding

Ingredients (for 1 serving):

✓ ¼ cup of chia seeds about 32g

✓ ¼ cup coconut milk or heavy whipped cream about 60ml

✓ ½ cup of almond milk or water about 120 ml

- ✓ 1/4 tsp of cinnamon

- ✓ 1 tbsp of Swerve or Erythritol about 10gms

- ✓ 5-10 drops of Stevia extract

- ✓ ½ cup of fresh or frozen berries about 38gms

Instructions:

1. Start by mixing the chia seeds, water, coconut milk, stevia, Erythritol and cinnamon. To get a smoother texture, place the mixture into a blender and pulse until it becomes smooth. Mix the berries and let that sit for 15 minutes in the fridge. You can even sit the mixture in the fridge overnight for better taste.

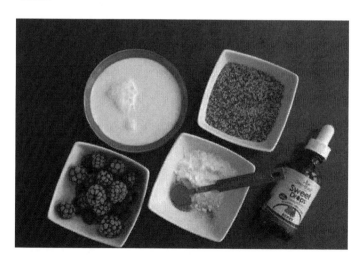

2. Take it out of the fridge and serve!

Lunch recipes

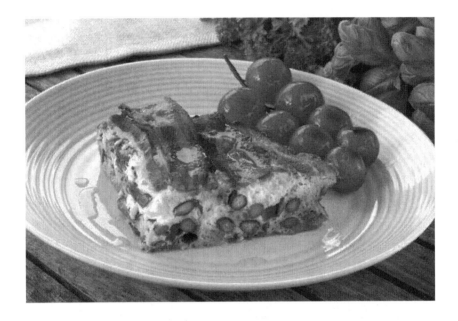

1. Easter Frittata

Ingredients (for 4 servings):

✓ 10 large eggs (organic or free-range)

✓ 20 small asparagus spears about 250gms

✓ 2 small spring onions about 10gms

✓ 1 small shallot about 20gms

✓ 1 red bell pepper about 150gms

✓ ¼ cup of full-fat cream about 60ml

✓ 1 package of fresh soft goat cheese or any other soft full fat cheese about 150gms

✓ 1 package of Pancetta or bacon about 100gms

✓ 2 tbsp of fresh parsley

✓ 2 tbsp of fresh mint

✓ 1 tbsp of fresh tarragon

✓ 2 tbsp of unsalted organic butter or ghee

✓ Salt and black pepper to taste

✓ 4 cherry tomato vines about 300gms

Instructions:

1. Start with preheating the oven up to 400 F. start preparing the asparagus by cutting off their woody ends. Wash and remove the seeds of the bell pepper and slice it into small stripes. Peel and then finely chop the spring onion and shallot.

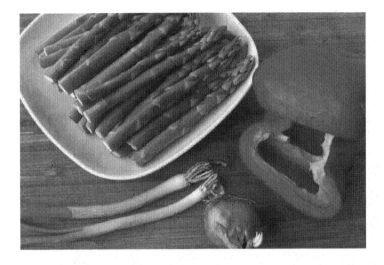

2. Use a tbsp of butter/ghee to grease the non-sticky pan, and add all the ingredients from the step above. Sprinkle some salt, and cook briefly for about 5 minutes till you get a good fragrance coming out of it. Turn off the heat and put it aside.

3. Whisk the eggs in a bowl, add cream and freshly chopped herbs to it, and whisk again. If you don't have the herbs mentioned in the ingredients, you can simply use common herbs like thyme, chives and basil. Then season with black pepper and salt.

5. Put all the cooked veggies into a baking dish. Crumble the goat cheese and sprinkle it equally over the veggies. After that, you have to pour the egg mixture over the vegetables.

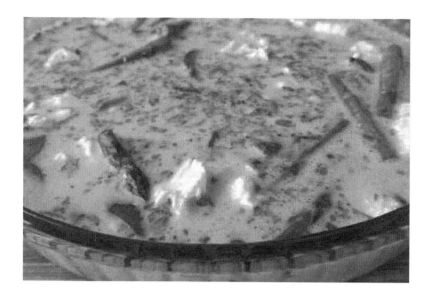

6. Place the baking dish into the oven and cook for about 20 minutes. Take it out when the top becomes firm.

7. Take the dish out of the oven carefully and reduce the oven's temperature to 350F. Lay the bacon or pancetta over the frittata, and put it back into the oven for another 15-20 minutes. When done, take it out of the oven, and wait till it cools down.

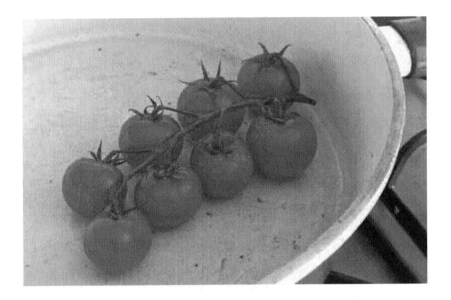

7. Meanwhile, you can prepare the tomatoes. Grease the pan with a tbsp of butter or ghee and keep the heat to a medium. The best way you can roast the tomatoes is by leaving the vines on. This will add additional flavor while you cook the tomatoes for about 5 minutes.

8. Serve the frittata with the tomatoes on the side!

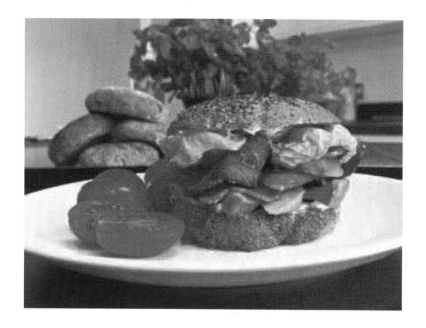

2. Keto Bun with Avocado & Bacon

Ingredients (for 1 serving):

- ✓ 1 Keto bun

- ✓ 2 tbsp of butter

- ✓ 2 small slices of bacon about 30gms

- ✓ ½ cherry tomatoes about 75gms

- ✓ ½ avocado about 100gm

- ✓ 2 leaves of fresh green lettuce

Instructions:

1. Start with cutting the bun in half and toast it till it takes a golden brown shade.

2. Splatter the buns with butter

3. Sauté the bacon till its crispy

4. Slice up the tomatoes and avocado

5. Place the lettuce, tomatoes, avocado and bacon between the two halves of buns, and get ready to take the first bite!

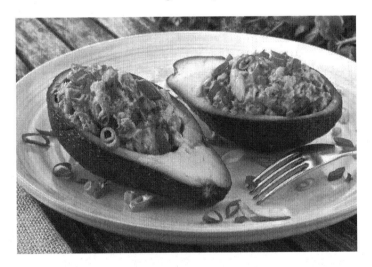

3. Paleo Styled Stuffed Avocado

Ingredients (for 1 serving):

✓　1 large avocado about 200gms

✓　1 tin of drained sardines about 90gms

✓　1 tbsp of mayonnaise about 15gms

✓　1 medium sized spring onion or a bunch of chives about 15gms

✓　Juice from ¼ of a lemon

✓　¼ tsp turmeric powder

✓　¼ tsp salt

Instructions:

1.　Start by cutting the avocado in halves and remove its seed. Drain the right amount of sardines and put them in a bowl.

2.　Scoop out the flesh of the avocado leaving only a ½ - 1 inch of flesh inside.

3.　Add finely sliced spring onion and sprinkle some turmeric powder. Then add the mayonnaise and mix the ingredients well.

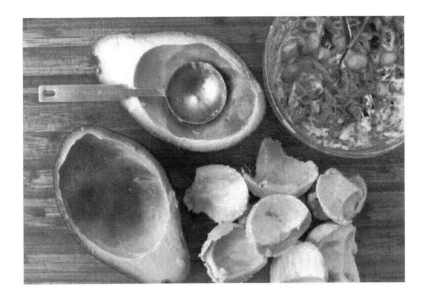

4. Take the scooped out avocado flesh and add to the mix, and mash it into the consistency you desire. Sprinkle some salt and squeeze some lemon juice.

5. Put the mixture into the avocado halves and get ready to enjoy!

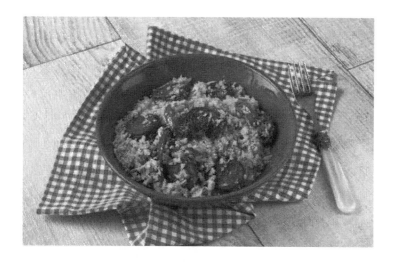

4. Keto Mexican Rice

Ingredients (for 4 servings):

✓ 5 cups Cauli-rice from about 1 average sized cauliflower about 600gms

✓ 2 pepperoni or Spanish chorizo sausages about 240gms

✓ 6 to 8 jalapeno peppers about 80gms

✓ 4 tbsp of freshly chopped cilantro or parsley

✓ 2 tbsp ghee, coconut oil or butter about 30gms

✓ Salt to taste

Instructions:

1. Prepare the cauli rice and make sure you don't overcook it.

2. Slice and deseed the jalapenos, and slice up the sausages. If jalapeno is too hot for you, go for other alternatives.

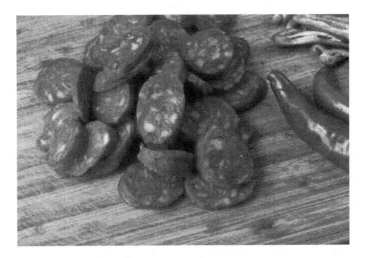

3. Use butter or ghee to grease a skillet, and sauté the peppers and sausage slices. Stir and cook until they are brown.

4. Add the cauliflower rice and keep cooking for about 5 to 10 minutes, depending on how tender you want the rice to be. Sprinkle some salt and then the chopped parsley over it.

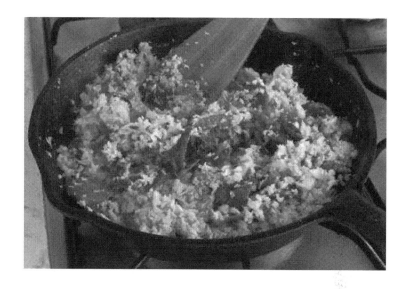

5. When cooked, turn off the heat and serve!

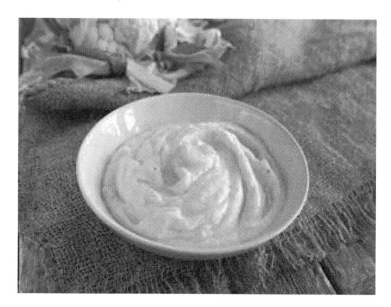

5. Pork Chops with Creamy Mash

Ingredients (for 1 serving)

✓ 1 medium pork chop about 150gms

✓ 1 tbsp of ghee or butter

✓ Salt and pepper

✓ 1 serving of creamy keto mash

Instructions:

1. Start by sautéing the pork chop with the 1 tbsp of butter or ghee, and season it with salt and pepper.

2. When cooked, turn off the heat and serve with 1 serving of creamy keto mash!

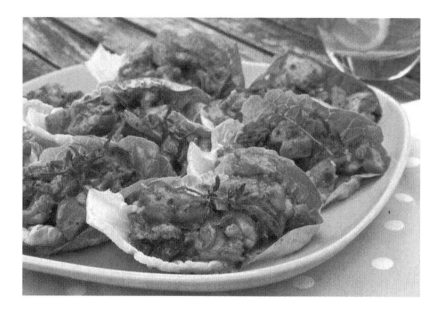

6. Cajun Chicken Tacos

Ingredients (for 2 servings):

✓   1 package of chicken thighs, boneless and skinned about 400gms

✓   ½ medium sized red onion about 50gms

✓   ½ lime juice

✓   2 cloves of garlic

✓   1 tbsp of fresh thymes

✓   1 tbsp of fresh oregano

✓   ½ tsp of paprika

- ✓ ½ tsp of cayenne pepper

- ✓ 2 tbsp of butter or ghee

- ✓ Fresh coconut milk or full fat cream about 60ml

- ✓ Salt and pepper

- ✓ 2 heads of small lettuce about 200gms

Instructions:

1. Peel and finely chop the onions and fresh herbs. And mash the garlic.

2. Dice all the chicken thighs, and marinate with herbs, garlic, cayenne, paprika, lime juice, salt and pepper.

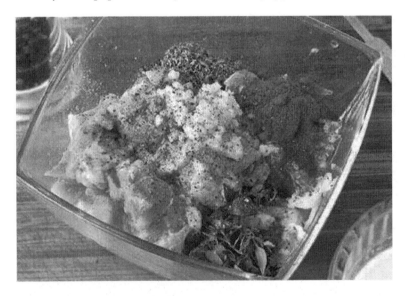

3. Heat up a large skillet and grease it with butter or ghee to cook the onions over medium heat. Stir till the onions become soft and golden brown.

4. Add the marinated chicken pieces and let it cook for about 10 minutes till the chicken is tender.

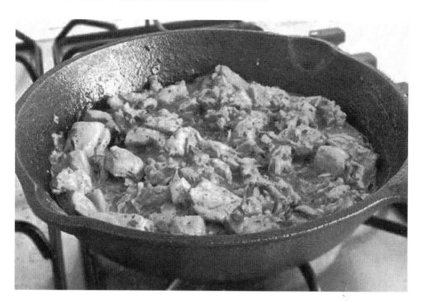

5. Keep the heat on medium and add the cream. Stir and let it cook for another 2 to 3 minutes. When done, turn off the heat and set aside the skillet.

6. Wash the lettuce and soak the water with a paper towel.

7. Scoop up the meat mixture, place it on top of the lettuce leafs, and get ready to serve!

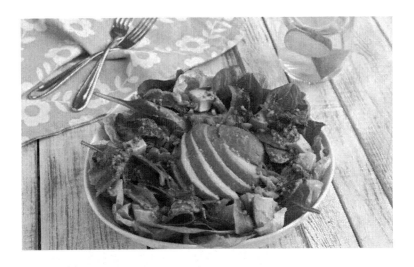

7. Avocado Salad

Ingredients (for 2 servings)

- ✓ 2 average sized avocados about 400gms

- ✓ 2 small heads of lettuce about 200gms

- ✓ 2 cups of fresh spinach about 60gms

- ✓ 1 medium sized spring onion about 15gms

- ✓ 4 large bacon slices about 120gms

- ✓ 2 sliced hard boiled eggs (optional)

Instructions:

1. Grease a skillet with bit of butter or ghee and heat it to fry the bacon

2. Meanwhile, tear the lettuce and wash the spinach. Use a salad spinner to dry the leaves.

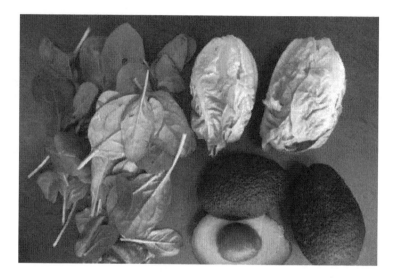

3. Cut the avocadoes in half and get rid of the seeds. Then slice them up in fine stripes.

4. Prepare the vinaigrette by mixing all the necessary ingredients.

5. Peel and slice up the hard boiled eggs (optional)

6. Fold the spinach and lettuce in a bowl and assemble the salad. Torn the crispy bacon in small pieces and sprinkle it all

over. Then put the sliced up avocadoes in the middle. Time to enjoy!

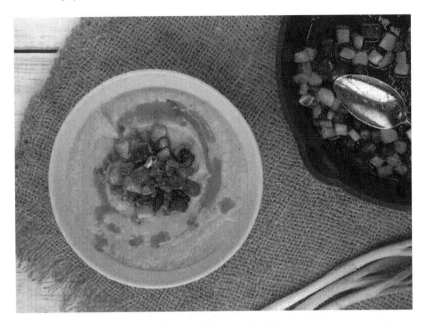

8. Spicy Cauliflower Soup

Ingredients (for 6 servings):

✓ 1 large cauliflower about 800gms

✓ 1 medium turnip about 200gms

✓ 1 small white onion about 70gms

✓ 2 cups of chicken stock about 480 ml

✓   1 medium sized pepperoni or Spanish chorizo sausage about 150 gms

✓   3 tbsp of butter or ghee about 45gms

✓   ½ tsp of salt

✓   Chives or 1 medium spring onion for garnishing about 15gms

Instructions:

1.   First off, wash the cauliflower and make small florets by cutting it.

2.   Get a soup pot and grease it with butter or ghee. Add the finely chopped onion and cook over medium heat for 5 minutes. Then add the chicken stock and cover the pot with a lid. Let it cook for about 10 minutes.

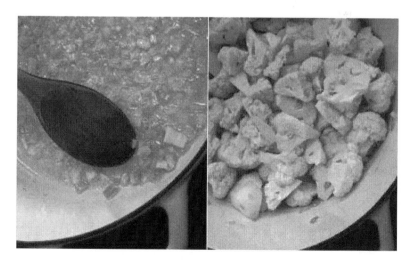

3.   Dice up the chorizo sausages. Peel and then finely dice the turnip. Place them on a heavy based skillet after greasing it with the remaining butter or ghee. Let it cook over medium heat until the sausage becomes crispy and the turnip becomes tender. It should take about 8 to 10 minutes.

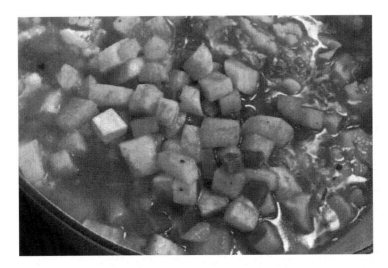

4.   Transfer the turnip and the sausage into the soup. Then use a hand blender to pulse the mixture into a smooth and creamy texture. Season the soup with cayenne pepper and salt. You can also add a cup of heavy whipped cream to add better taste.

5.   Pour the soup into the serving bowl and sprinkle some more turnip and chorizo mixture, and then drizzle some of that spicy oil. Use the freshly chopped spring onion or chives for garnishing, and get ready to serve!

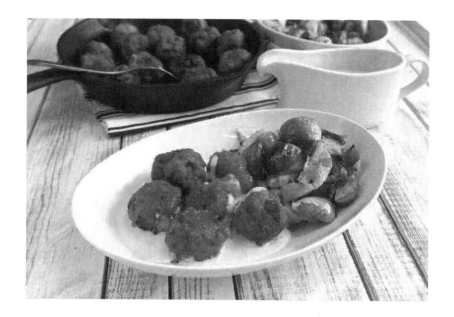

9. Spicy Chorizo Meatballs

Ingredients (for 4 servings):

- ✓ 0.9 lb of ground pork about 400gms

- ✓ ⅓ of average sized Spanish chorizo sausage about 80gms

- ✓ 1 large egg

- ✓ ½ cup of almond flour about 50gms

- ✓ 1 tsp paprika

- ✓ ¼ tsp of cayenne pepper

- ✓ 1 tsp of ground cumin

✓   2 cloves of garlic

✓   1 small sized white onion about 70gms

✓   1 tbsp ghee

✓   Salt to taste

Instructions:

1.   Start by peeling and dicing the garlic, onion and chorizo sausages.

2.   Use the ghee to grease a large pan and put over medium heat. Add the chorizo, onion and garlic and cook for 5 to 8 minutes till the ingredients become lightly crisp. Take the heat off and put the pan aside.

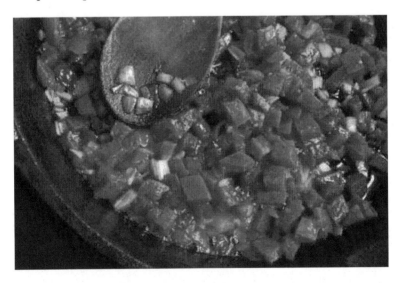

3. Get a mixing bowl and combine the egg, ground pork, paprika, almond flour, ground cumin, salt and cayenne pepper. Keep mixing until it becomes soft dough. Add the crisped up chorizo, onion and garlic into it and mix again.

4. Create small balls of the mixture using your hands, and place it on a cutting board.

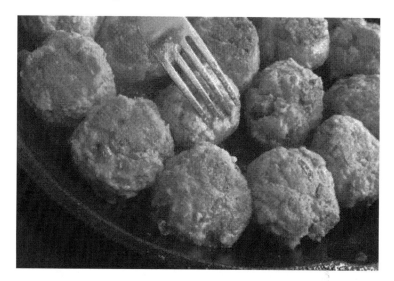

5. Heat the same pan you used for frying the chorizo to cook the meatballs until it becomes golden brown. Use a fork to turn the meatballs so that all the sides are properly cooked. It should take about 5 to 10 minutes, depending on the size of the meatballs.

6. Once ready, turn off the heat and serve immediately!

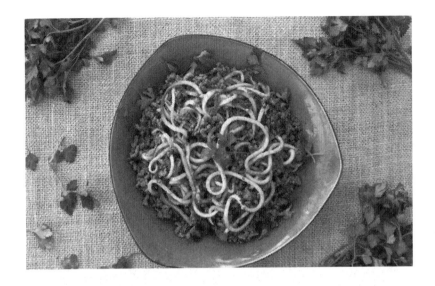

10.   Beef Ragù with "Zoodles"

Ingredients (for 4 servings):

✓   Grass-fed, minced beef about 800gms

✓   ¼ cup of red pesto about 65gms

✓   4 medium sized zucchinis

✓   1 tbsp of butter or ghee (herb or garlic infused for additional flavor)

✓   Bunch fresh parsley

✓   Salt

Instructions:

1. Make the "zoodle" by slicing the zucchini using a vegetable peeler and spiralizer.

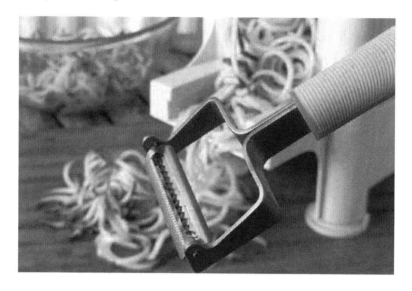

2. Grease a sauce pan with ghee and place the meat in it. If you are using frozen meat, make you keep defrost it before cooking. Cook the meat until it is brown from all the sides. You would also have to keep stirring. It should take about 5 to 8 minutes to cook.

3. Add the freshly chopped parsley and red pesto and keep the mixture on low heat. When you take it off the heat, transfer it into a bowl.

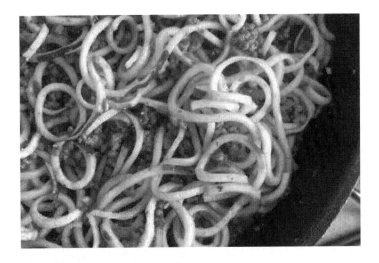

4. Transfer the zoodles into a saucepan, which you need to grease first with the remaining ghee. Cook the zoodles for about 3-5 minutes. Turn off the heat and add the meat in the zoodles. Cook it till the zoodles become soft.

5. Turn off the heat and serve!

Dinner recipes

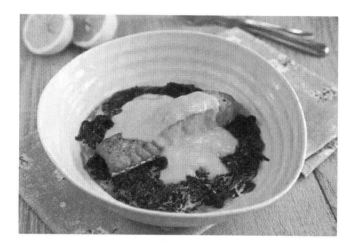

1. Salmon with Creamy Spinach & Hollandaise Sauce

Ingredients (for 1 serving):

- ✓ 1 small fillet of salmon or trout about 125gms

- ✓ ½ large packet of fresh or frozen spinach

- ✓ 1 tbsp of heavy whipped cream

- ✓ 2 tbsp of coconut oil or ghee

- ✓ 1 serving of Hollandaise sauce

- ✓ Ground black pepper

- ✓ Salt

Instructions:

1. Preheat the oven up to 400 F. drizzle a baking tray with coconut oil or ghee, and place the salmon in it. Season the fish with pepper and salt and place the tray inside the oven. Cook for around 20 to 25 minutes.

2. Meanwhile, prepare the spinach by washing it and placing it on a salad spinner to get rid of the excess water.

   Grease a skillet with ghee and put it over medium heat. Cook the spinach for 3 to 5 minutes while stirring. Season it with salt.

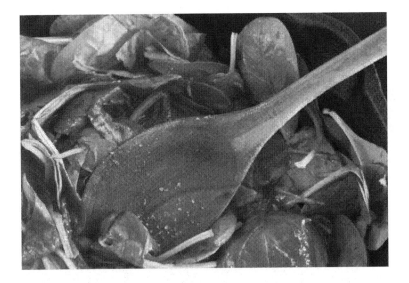

3. Add coconut milk or heavy whipped cream.

4. Take it off the heat and prepare the Hollandaise sauce.

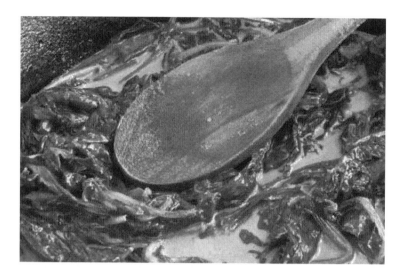

5.   Take the salmon out of the oven and set it aside.

6.   Place the creamy spinach on a serving plate and place the salmon on top of it.

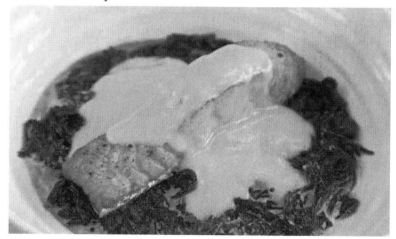

7.   Pour Hollandaise sauce over it and it is ready to being served!

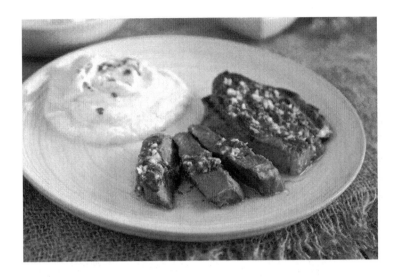

2. Ribeye Steak with Gremolata

Ingredients (for 2 servings)

- ✓ 2 small grass fed ribeye steaks about 400gms

- ✓ ¼ salts

- ✓ Freshly ground black pepper

- ✓ 4 tbsp of freshly chopped parsley

- ✓ 2 cloves of garlic

- ✓ 2 tsp of freshly grated organic lemon zest

- ✓ 3 tbsp of ghee or extra virgin olive oil

Instructions:

1. Let the steak to sit at room temperature for about 10 to 15 minutes. Use a paper towel to soak the excess blood. Pour some melted ghee over it and season the meat with pepper and salt. Ghee tends to solidify even in room temperature and that is completely normal.

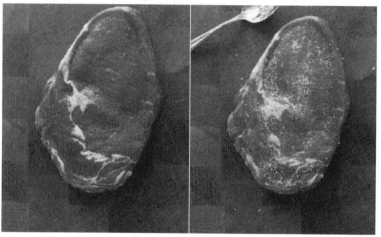

2. Make the Gremolata by mixing melted ghee with mashed garlic, chopped parsley, and finely grated lemon zest. Season it with salt and set aside for later. When using ghee, keep the Gremolata warm or the ghee will solidify.

3. Place a heavy based pan over high heat and fry the steak keeping each side down for 2 to 4 minutes. When the sides will turn brown, flip the steak over. Depending on the size of your steak, it may take about 5 minutes to cook completely.

Reduce the heat to a medium and cook for another 11 minutes. You won't need to turn the steak once you reduce the temperature to medium.

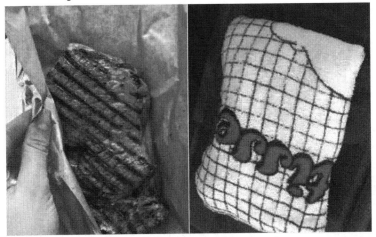

4. Once cooked, get the steak out of the pan and allow it to rest in a warm place for 5 to 7 minutes. During this period, the steak will cook on residual heat. The best idea is to keep the steak covered in brown paper and then wrap it in a towel. This will keep the steak juicy and pink inside.

5. Slice the steak and serve it on the place with Gremolata and keto cream mash on the side. Enjoy!

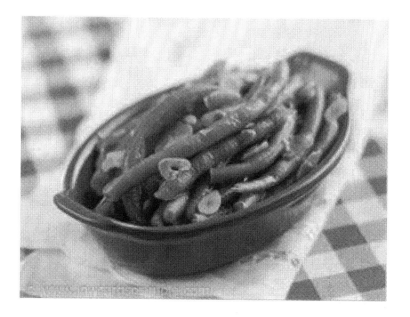

3. Pan-roasted salmon with green beans

Ingredients:

- ✓ 1 medium fillet of salmon about 150gms

- ✓ 1 serving of lemon juice

- ✓ Salt

- ✓ Pepper

- ✓ Lemon juice

Instructions:

1. Grease a pan with ghee and fry the salmon fillet. Season it with lemon juice, pepper and salt.

2. Serve the fish with 1 serving of green beans. Then sprinkle chopped almonds, and add a dash of lemon juice before serving.

Chapter 8

WRAPPING UP

A lot has been said about the ketogenic diet. We have discussed all the different aspects of how ketosis starts and how you can adapt to this unconventional yet uniquely healthy lifestyle. Despite all the debate that prevails regarding ketogenic, it can be said with certainty that this diet is accompanied by some great benefits. If you are looking forward to achieving your desired weight and leading a healthy life, this low carb and high fat diet can help you make your dreams come true! If you have been eyeing that dress for ages, but haven't gotten the courage to buy it simply because you fear it won't fit you, it is time you begin your keto journey. Few months into the keto lifestyle, and you will start noticing the significant improvements that it will bring your body and overall health.

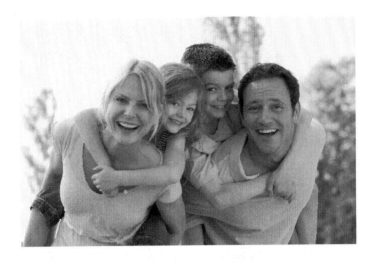

If you are suffering from various diseases like epilepsy and diabetes, and want to put an end to the constant troubles that come with them, start learning how you can benefit from a state of ketosis. A ketogenic diet may be able to do what medicines have failed so far. All you have to do is keep an open mind, and give this diet an honest and fair chance. What have you got to lose? On any given day, you are going to benefit from this revolutionary diet. So, consult your physician or nutritionist about options you have as far as adapting to the keto lifestyle is concerned. Also, gather as much knowledge as you can about this diet and how it affects your particular situation. When you approach this diet armed with sufficient knowledge, there will be no room for error. So, if you are ready to lead a healthy balanced diet, swear by this low carb, high fat/protein diet!

Hey,

If you liked this book, them I'm happy☺

My hope is that it helped you in some way.

If you'd like to learn more about my other books, check out the info below: http://www.amazon.com/Valerie-Childs/e/B00VVS8TYO

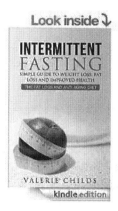

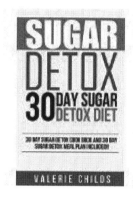

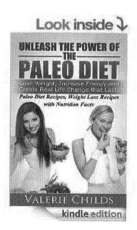

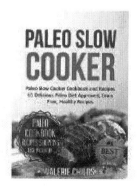

Conclusion

Thank you again for downloading this book!

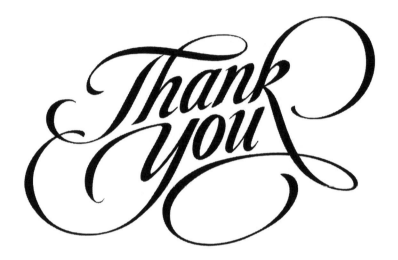

If you enjoyed this book, then I'd like to ask you for a favor, would you be kind enough to leave a review for this book on Amazon? It'd be greatly appreciated!

Help us better serve you by sending questions or comments to greatreadspublishing@gmail.com - Thank you!

Made in the USA
San Bernardino, CA
07 March 2017